Closed World
of
Love

ARCHIE HILL

SIMON AND SCHUSTER · NEW YORK

DESIGNED BY EVE METZ.
MANUFACTURED IN THE UNITED STATES OF AMERICA

1 2 3 4 5 6 7 8 9 10
LIBRARY OF CONGRESS CATALOGING IN PUBLICATION
DATA

HILL, ARCHIE.
    CLOSED WORLD OF LOVE.

        1. PARALYSIS, SPASTIC—BIOGRAPHY.   2. CHIL-
DREN, ADOPTED—BIOGRAPHY.   3. HILL, BARRY.
4. LOVE, PATERNAL.   5. STEPFATHERS—BIOGRAPHY.
6. HILL, ARCHIE.   I. TITLE.
RJ496.S6H54   301.42'7 [B]   77-3048
ISBN 0-671-22845-5

THIS SMALL BOOK
IS MY WAY OF
EXPRESSING MY LOVE
AND THANKS TO
BARRY,
ROBIN,
AND ESPECIALLY
MY WIFE.

Contents

1

A Shadow
in the Room's Corner

HE WAS FOURTEEN years old when I first met him, a wee little thin chap living in a wheelchair, who couldn't speak or walk, but I remember how his eyes were warm with deep intelligence. His eyes were the main thing I remembered about him. Rich warm brown, like his mother's. He seemed more like a six or seven years' old child than a fourteen. Small and light of bone, he was no more than a shadow in the room's corner if you didn't look at him direct. I seldom deliberately looked at him in those early days—it was his mother I looked at, because she I was in love with, and her son was merely a shadow-image at the edge of her life which had no claim on my attention.

I was living in a one-room setup in North London. A bed, a drunken-door wardrobe, a cane-bottomed chair, a small washbasin, and an electric-element cooker made up my home. The house was rent-shared by sixteen other people, mostly West Indians, and owned by a Greek. The electric cooker was the worst thing in my room—it ate the shillings up and took its time in making anything warm, let alone cooked. I estimated that the element took half an hour to boil a two-cup kettle, and at weekends—when I ate in—it was necessary to start cooking lunch at breakfast time so that it could be eaten at tea time.

But even so, the one-room setup was the first "home" I'd had in a good many years, other than doss houses, Sally-Army hostels and sleeping rough. Two years behind me was a prison discharge, and I'd come to London either to lose my identity or find another; and I didn't seem to be getting anywhere at all. Just drifting and floating, trying to find some roots I could name as my own. Most of my after-work hours seemed to be spent in public houses, matching glass for glass with other bed-sitter types who'd equally got no roots.

I used to think, "One day I shall step outside myself . . . one day I shall look back on what I could have been and will never have known myself. Telescope or microscope, I will never have known myself."

At the time I was doing a variety of jobs, all casual and impermanent. For a spell I'd been a gravedigger, which didn't last very long. When a man has started to come back to life he doesn't want to be surrounded by the dead. I'd worked on building sites, as a door-to-door seller of cleaning brushes, as a painter and decorator swinging high in a cradle on the flanks of near-skyscrapers. Months went by. On the outside I was normal. On the inside I was empty. Going through motions. No purpose, no ambition. Just working, drinking, mixing with floaters and drifters. . . .

And then, to supplement my earnings, I got a Saturday job in a furniture store—as a "humper," not as a salesman. I just had to "hump" furniture around the salesrooms or to the delivery vans. And this lovely woman came into the store to buy a wardrobe. All the salesmen were busy with customers, and it was part of my job in such cases to keep a potential customer engaged until a salesman could come across. I took this beautiful woman on a tour of inspection of wardrobes and I didn't know maple from walnut, oak from mahogany—which fact seemed to amuse her. Neither could I get any of the door keys to work, which seemed to amuse her more. She didn't laugh openly but I could see the laughter in her eyes, and it made me feel warm. She decided on a particular style of wardrobe but we hadn't got the color grain she wanted in stock. So I took a deposit from her and made out an order invoice, telling her it would need about a week's waiting for the goods to arrive. I wrote her name on the invoice with disappointment: "Mrs." She was married . . . just my luck. And I'd felt so close with her, emotionally close, while we were walking round the showrooms. Closer than I'd felt with anybody for a long, long time. Not being able to place my accent, she asked me where I came from, and I said "the Black Country," then protested when she said, "Oh, Birmingham." "The Black Country's not Birmingham," I told her. "It's a separate place altogether. I come from half a stone's toss from Shropshire." And that lovely smile of hers, warming her mouth and eyes.

"Housman," she said. "You *look* like his Shropshire Lad."

Which I thought was a very nice compliment.

During the next several weeks she haunted me on two fronts. One, the wardrobe didn't arrive from the warehouse and I had to lie to her, making one excuse after another. Two . . . she just haunted me. But the title "Mrs." stood between my thoughts and my mouth and wouldn't let me try to date her. Every Saturday she called by. I think eventually she didn't call to see if the wardrobe had arrived but merely to confirm that it hadn't. She told me that she wanted it for a spare room in her house that she'd decided to make into a bed-sitter and let to some single person.

One Saturday night, after I'd spent several hours in the pub, I sat in my room and its threadbare ugliness hit me like a clenched fist. My bits of gear were spread all around. Clothing in the built-in cupboard, toothbrush and razor on the sink ledge, couple of pipes in the soup dish which served as ashtray. Possessions, but no roots. No roots anywhere. Tinny music blared from some West Indian's room, kids were playing and shrilling in the streets, and god I felt lonely and dried up and empty and sick inside my mind. On top of which I was in love with a married woman.

Next morning, Sunday, I walked round to her

house. My heart was pumping what for as I rang the front doorbell, and suddenly I was scared as a kid and wanted to run away—what if her husband, at least six feet high and weighing a hundred and eighty pounds, confronted me and read my eyes? I could hear his voice thundering in my imagination: "What the hell you mean, you're in love with my wife?"

She opened the door.

"The Shropshire Lad," she said, warm-smiling. "Don't tell me you've brought the wardrobe on a handcart?"

"I've come about the room," I blurted, "the one you said you're going to let."

She opened the door wide.

"Come in," she said. "I've just made a fresh pot of tea."

It was about eleven o'clock in the morning when I went in; it was near midnight when I left. I had lunch there, tea and supper. With her, her widowed mother and bachelor brother.

And Barry.

I hardly noticed Barry . . . he was just a child in a wheelchair, no more. Except his eyes, and they were brown and warm as his mother's.

"Where's your husband?" I asked, making my voice polite and neutral.

"We're divorced," she answered, and I swear my head rang with bell music and a symphony orchestra started up somewhere in my gut, and the birds singing in the trees outside came up with a conspiracy of rare harmony, every one of 'em in tune with each other and not competing. And I swear the flowers on the window ledge in their cut-glass vase took on five dimensions of color and I could smell their scent from ten feet off. The tea I was drinking suddenly tasted like fresh honey taken from the hive. "I'm divorced as well," I said.

She took me upstairs to the spare room.

"I shall have to decorate it before I let it," she said.

"I'll do it," I jumped in quickly, "I'm a pretty good decorator."

She was doubtful.

"We'd really planned on letting to a girl," she said. "You know—a nurse or a student. We'd really planned on having a girl in."

Dismay filled me.

"It's a miserable place I'm living in," I told her. "It's so damned miserable it's almost impossible. I could make this into a nice room—I wouldn't get in your way."

She led me back downstairs.

"Whoever we let to," she explained, "would have to take meals with us. There'd be no cooking arrangements in the room. Our lodger would have to eat with the family."

"I'm not a fussy eater," I gabbled. "I eat anything that's put in front of me—and I don't smoke in bed—and I wipe my feet on the mat when I come in off the street. . . ."

"We'll see," she answered. "We'll think about it."

Back in my Greek-room about an hour after midnight I wrote her a letter. I gabbled on about what a nice day she and her family had given me, how I'd love to decorate the spare room and move in and p.s. would she come to the pictures with me on Wednesday evening. I'd collect her at her front door at six o'clock.

We went to the pictures. I don't recall what the film was about or who was in it. I only remember the box of chocolates I bought for her. I don't normally eat chocolates. But she sat with the open box on her lap in the cinema darkness, and every now and then when I saw from the corner of my eye that she was lifting one out I took one too, so's my hand could accidentally touch hers.

I asked her to come for a drink, once we were outside the cinema.

"No," she answered, "I must go home."

"It's early yet."

"I must get home. I have Barry to see to."

"Barry? Oh—the boy."

"I must get back to him and feed him, then get him ready for bed."

I walked her home.

"Will I see you again?" I asked.

She smiled.

"If you still want to be our lodger, you'll not be off seeing me," she said.

I was as happy as a kid with a birthday gift.

"You mean—I can move in?"

"You'll have to decorate the room first."

"When?"
"Whenever you like."
"Tomorrow?"
"If you like."
"I like," I said. "Oh, yes—I like."

Four nights later, the decorating finished, I moved in . . . and planted my roots.

2

Building Blocks

WHEN I ASKED HER to marry me, she was serious, solemn. A strange withdrawn look about her, as if reliving some experience, some memory, that was not of me.

"Would you want children?" she asked at last, and I shrugged.

"One or two, perhaps," I said, "but one would be all right."

Sadness in her eyes.

"No," she said. "I can't marry you."

"Can't? Or won't?"

"I can't. I have Barry—he needs me."

"*I* need you."

Dark eyes on mine.

"You are fit and healthy. Barry isn't. He needs me more."

I puzzled at it.

"You can't go through life on your own," I said. "You need a man. You're young—and I can be on hand to look after Barry. He's only a wee chap, he's no trouble at all."

"He won't always remain small. He'll grow.

He'll need me more and more as he grows older."

I thought about it, then let my mind shrug its shoulders.

"I'm not bothered about children," I said at last. "It doesn't matter if I don't have a child . . . I'll make Barry my child."

Her face softened, the warm and radiant beauty came back.

"Think about it," she said, "and tell me when you are sure."

"I'm sure now," I answered. "Children of my own don't matter. You couldn't look after Barry as well—I don't want any children."

So we were married soon after.

I used to watch her with him, him so small and thin. Every night for a couple of hours she'd take him from his wheelchair and lay him out on the floor, then massage his limbs and exercise him. She'd got this big mirror which she used to lean against the wall so Barry could see himself being exercised. She'd make a game of it with him. Then she got two lengths of wood, the same size and shape as snow skis. At the front end she fastened a pair of Barry's shoes; and at the back end she fastened a pair of her own. She'd slip her feet and his into the shoes, hold him under the armpits, and start walking. The movement of her own legs caused the "skis" to act like pistons, making Barry's legs go through the motions of walking. I watched her do this year in and year out . . . but no good came of it. Barry never learned how to walk.

22

During the evening hours I used to watch her with him. She'd prop him comfortably on the sofa, sit alongside him, and try to get his fingers to manipulate building blocks with pictures on them. Hour after hour she'd sit with him, calm, serene, never impatient.

It was I who grew impatient.

"Let's put him to bed," I'd say, "and go out for a bit. Your mum will look after him for us."

And sometimes she'd do just that. But if we were at the cinema or having a meal someplace I'd see her eyes ever glancing at her wristwatch, and I'd know her thoughts were with Barry back home. He'd be waiting to be spoonfed his last meal of the day, for his teeth to be cleaned, his body to be sponge-bathed, his nappy to be changed. Long tied routines waiting to be done each and every day. Sometimes I felt stabs of jealousy against the boy because he was taking more of his mother's attention than I was. When she was with him, I felt as if I stood in second place. And I wanted always to be in first place.

When I became aware of this jealousy I tried to destroy it, to get it out of my system. I'd clown around for him, try to make him laugh—actions of entertainment prompted by my own guilt, I think. Guilt for the feelings of ambivalence I sometimes had for him, when he was taking all of his mother's attention and leaving none for me. He was, I think, still very much of a room-shadow that sometimes blocked out the light. But I tried to accept him,

23

tried to come to terms with the fact that he'd got to share his life with us, and I'd got to share my life with him because I was sharing his mother.

We'd got a budgie and one day it laid a tiny egg. When his mother boiled eggs for breakfast, she usually spooned one into Barry's mouth. But this time when she'd got the eggs ready I took the budgie egg, painted a small clown's face on to its surface with inks, then placed it in a thimble instead of an egg cup. Barry's face was a picture of astonishment as he looked at it in front of him, and then the puppet-movement of his head, like a doll with awkwardly articulated joints, as he looked at the real eggs in front of his mother and myself. The sudden laughter flushing his face . . . making him appear normal, and lovely . . .

I watched her spoonfeeding food into him, egg and bread and milk whipped into a paste so that it would go into his mouth easily and without choking him. The paste oozed from the corners of his mouth and she scooped it back with the spoon-bowl. Slow, slow. She so patient, serene and gentle. (Where is the Rodin or Michelangelo who could sculpture such patience and love in all its truth?)

I'd never met love like it before—my ideas of love had been so shallow, so self-centered. What privileged few among us really know what love is? We know self-love, pride-love, power-love, money-love, comfort-love, dependent-love. We know shallow-love and glitter-love and love by many other

24

names; we know man-woman love which, as time passes and youth with it, turns into the safety of comfortable habit. There are good and rich loves, too, but there are different levels and depths of love and the deepest depth of all is this closed world of love which exists between a mother and the helpless creature which was the child drawn in pain from her body into a poisoned light of day.

Early in our marriage I was working as a jobbing builder. I wasn't enjoying the work, but the house-keeping money was coming in.

"I want to talk to you," my wife said, calm and practical—not lecturing or nagging. Helping me.

"I fell in love with you because of your mind," she said, "because of the contents of your mind—and you're not doing justice to yourself."

I was disturbed and puzzled.

"You mean you're not satisfied with me just being a workman?" I asked her. "Wearing overalls and getting my hands dirty?"

"You know I don't mean that at all. I respect the way you work—but I think you have better things in you, and you won't let them come out."

"What should I do, then? I've no qualifications in any direction."

"There are libraries. There are evening classes . . . you can take any direction you choose."

"What do you want me to do, then?"

She shook her head.

"No—it's not what *I* want you to do. I'm happy

for you to be doing anything that *you're* happy doing . . . but you're not happy."

"I'll think about which road," I answered. "I'll think on it."

I changed jobs a dozen times. This and that. Cutting cloth in a tailoring shop, packing cartons in a warehouse, a bit of clerical work. None of it attracted me.

She bought Barry a new bed, a cot bed, and I went into the garden shed and fetched tins of paint out, hunted around for a kid's camel-hair painting brush. With Barry watching, I painted pictures on the headboard of his new bed. Bambi-deer—a mom, dad and baby deer. And round them, in paint, I planted a forest and a pool for them to drink from. She and Barry watched the picture grow.

"It's lovely," my wife said. "It's really beautiful." She looked at me long and solemn.

"You *are* wasting your time," she said, "you really are. You have so much in you."

Barry's eyes were round with wonder. Little noises of pleasure came from his throat, little bleatings of wonder as he saw the picture come out of the brush.

Time went by. Evenings and weekends I was happy enough, because I was home. Home. What a wonderful word. . . .

But I wasn't happy at work. Everything I worked at seemed surrounded by deadness and monotony, with no ambition attached to it. Zombie work, and what *she'd* said—"You have so much in you"—

kept niggling inside my mind. How could I please her?

I wrote a short story. When I'd finished it (my first!) I thought it very, very good; but I stuck it away in a drawer and forgot about it, and when I *did* come across it again and reread it, I thought, "No . . . you have no talent."

Then I came home from work one day, and there was a letter propped up on the shelf, addressed to me from the BBC.

My wife kept looking at the envelope and then at me. She seemed on tenterhooks.

"Aren't you going to open it?"

I kept turning the envelope round and round in my hands, wondering what on earth the BBC had written to me about. I opened the envelope and couldn't believe my eyes.

"The BBC," I blurted. "They've accepted that short story I wrote. They want to pay me for it and put it over the air—this is a contract." I kept staring at the letter and the contract, marveling at them. Then a thought struck me.

"Hey," I said, "what's happened? *I* never sent the story off—it's still in the drawer upstairs."

"*I* sent it," my wife answered. She set my tea on the table, sat opposite me.

"Do you see?" she asked me, and I nodded.

"Yes," I answered, "I do see."

"So what shall you do?"

"I shall learn to be a writer," I answered. "I'll keep at it until I win."

Her eyes were very warm.

"Yes," she said softly, "I hoped that's what you'd say."

I could tell from her face that her thoughts were picking a delicate direction for her words to walk along.

"I've some little savings," she said at last, "not a lot, but enough to tide us over for a year."

"What do you mean?"

"That you start straight away. Start writing, I mean. We can manage for a bit."

I thought about it for a while.

"Yes," I said at last, "I'd like to do it—do you think I can?"

She pointed to the letter.

"The BBC's given you the evidence you need," she said.

"But what do *you* think?"

"I don't *think* you can do it," she answered. "I *know* you can."

That year I wrote five more stories and three radio plays. They were all accepted. I worked in our bedroom, with ten pounds worth of second-hand typewriter whose return carriage broke down after the second short story was finished. I made it work again by incorporating a thick elastic band into its mechanism ... and life was many-splendored except for one small dark spot ever coming into my mind.

"Give me a child," I said to her, my wife. "I want a son of my own."

Her eyes were dark and sad on mine.

"We agreed not," she answered. "It would take me away from Barry. I couldn't cope. You said a child wouldn't matter."

I was restless.

"It didn't matter then," I said, "but lately, it seems to matter more and more. I'm in my mid-thirties and I keep wanting a child of my own."

She went shopping, leaving me to tend Barry. He'd become very real in my life; he'd stopped being a mere shadow. I sat looking at him, seeing his mother's face shining out from his; but I felt resentment toward him growing.

"Why do you have to be?" I asked him heavily. "Why do you have to get in the way of real life? Why don't you die and make room for others?" His eyes, like his mother's, were solemn on mine . . . almost as if he understood my words. Perhaps he did . . . we'd only got the doctor's word for it that he couldn't understand anything.

"You do understand, don't you?" I said. "You're not my son—you're another man's son. Why won't *he* come and take you away?"

His face was grave at the tone of my voice; showing no understanding of the words, only realizing there was no laughter in my voice. His head was angled to one side, puppetlike. He seemed so frail and vulnerable . . . and his eyes were his mother's eyes looking at me.

I felt a great surge of pity. I went to him, lifted him from his wheelchair, and carried him into the bedroom to change his nappy, which was wet and un-comfortable.

"Poor little bugger," I said to him. "It's not your fault you got short-changed at birth." His face laughed up at me, his senses recognizing the change in my voice. I took the wet nappy from him, put it into a bowl for washing, put a clean nappy on him. I fastened it with a huge safety pin taken from the dresser, not being able to find the smaller pin I'd taken from him. I dressed him clumsily, big bunches of clothing hunched and lumped around his body. I tried to squeeze and smooth the lumps out as you might do with dough on a pastry board. I picked him up and put him back into his wheel-chair, placed a new bib around his throat to catch his dribbles of mouth moisture.

"I'm going to have me a child of my own," I said to him, "come hell or high water. But don't you worry—you'll still be safe here with us. We won't throw you out on your ears."

When she conceived my child, I felt unease which grew almost into an obsession. Could she cope with the double responsibility? Had she enough of herself to give? Would, after all, a twisted ugly Fate duplicate the errors of Barry in the new life yet to come? Would the new life too cause heartbreak instead of heart-joy? . . . The si-lent questions I asked myself were endless and turmoiled. Compulsively and neurotically I delved and sifted into my wife's family history, its mem-

bers' lives and healths . . . looking for some malignant physical darkness which might be inherited,
passed on to the yet unborn child I so desperately
wanted. I felt utter loneliness within me. I couldn't
discuss it with anybody, my wife particularly, in
case I frightened her with my own fears. I tried
talking about it with medical "experts," but their
answers were vague, general, couched in terms
beyond my understanding. Phrases technical and
uncomforting. Twice, in panic and without con-
sulting my wife, I made enquiries about abortion.
All the time I believed these distressing anxieties
were private to me alone; but later I learned that
she too had been experiencing the same fears for
the duration of her pregnancy, but with deeper
pain because it was her body which carried my unborn son.

She was eight months pregnant and we were
putting a new mortise lock onto the back door.
I'd got mallet and wood chisel, pecking out a hole
in the leading edge of the door for the lock to fit
into. She was holding the door firm for me with her
hands, bracing it against my working blows . . . and
the door slipped, the wood chisel went off at a
tangent before I could regain my balance, drove its
cutting edge at her swollen belly. I saw her hands
clasp at the chisel blade, saw the blood pouring out.
Reality receded to the size of a pinprick. I felt
horror killing me, paralyzing my mind . . . I could
see the blood pouring from between her fingers
clasped to her belly, and then I could feel the sick-

ness wrenching the lining of my own stomach loose. And she was calm and unalarmed, quiet and soothing, talking me back to even keel.

"It's all right," I heard her saying from across chasms of space and time. "It's my hand is cut, nothing more."

There was a terrible gash along the palm of one hand. She'd reacted without thinking, reflexes faster than the speed of light, and caught the glancing chisel before it could penetrate her. I sat down, sick and weak, trembling head to foot. Then pulled myself together and dressed her wound.

She was always calm; that was the way of her. Calm and serene, tapping personal reservoirs of serenity that I never knew existed. I used to ask myself at what power plug did she recharge her emotional batteries. I knew that I could recharge mine from her: but where did (where does) she recharge hers? It is a mystery greater than man's triumphant trip to the moon and back, a mystery greater than my ability to comprehend. If God there is, then God is a woman: and if God isn't, then God should be. What do men like me know about creation? Nothing. We are no more than a tube of toothpaste which squirts a substance, and that's that. We are discardable containers where procreation is concerned—dispensable. Only the female of the species is indispensable if life is to go on—a sperm bank could last as long as earth will.

As the final stages of her pregnancy drew near I found myself becoming more and more tense. I know she sensed this, however hard I tried to hide it from her.

"Hush yourself," she'd tell me. "Everything is going to be all right." As she got heavier with carrying my child, I had to help out with Barry more and more. Lifting and carrying him . . . I couldn't point to the exact moment in time when I "accepted" him completely as mine; it just came about that way. The fact that he was not of my blood never seemed to trouble me anymore. His mother was my wife, and he was my son. I was often clumsy with him, I suppose, not having the same gentleness in my hands that his mother had. But there was gentleness for him in my mind, so I suppose that may have made up for a lot.

It was just after breakfast on a Sunday when she told me to fetch the ambulance, that our baby was coming. I'd had her suitcase packed for a week or so, and pennies put in a little dish for phoning the ambulance. I dashed out of the house to get to the street telephone, remembered I'd forgotten the pennies, and ran back for them. Back to the phone booth to make the call.

"Come straight away," I said into the mouthpiece. "My wife has started labor pains." I was hanging the piece back on to its rests when the firm, soothing, unhurried practical, disembodied voice of the operator stopped me.

"Give me the name and address before you hang up."

"O Lord," I thought, "I'm a right twit." I gave

the address, went back home. When the ambulance came I took my wife out to it, helped her inside. Then hammered on the sides of the ambulance to tell the driver to stop while I went back into the house for the suitcase.

When we got into the hospital, she sat on the bed and looked at me.

"There," she said softly, "that wasn't too bad, was it?" There was laughter in her voice and eyes the same as when I couldn't get the wardrobe keys to fit, the first day we ever met. I felt warm towards her.

"It'll be hours yet," she said, with nurses coming into the room to fuss her into bed, "so go home for a while, and look after Barry for me."

He was born at two-thirty that afternoon. My son. I went to her and him, but only she was there in the bed. I felt weight crushing me inside—surely my son should be there with her, in the bed? Surely they'd only take him away from her if there was something wrong with him . . . ? I tried to read her eyes. They were tired but happy—but was the look of happiness just put on while she prepared me for the worst? If he's not fit, I thought, let him be dead before I look at him. Don't let him be alive.

A nurse came in carrying this tiny wrinkled baby and held it out for me to see. I wouldn't touch him, my hands couldn't touch him. Not while a stranger held him. The nurse laid him in my wife's arms and went away—then I looked at him.

"Is he—is he—all right?" I asked my wife.

34

"He's beautiful.'

"Are you sure?"

"See for yourself." She opened the clothes from him as if they were petals opening from a rose to show the loveliness of its innermost core. I looked at my son, put my hands on him, letting my hands and eyes search for some grossness, some disability . . . and there he was, bawling and perfect and wholesome and complete. No blemish. No handicap. No imperfection in the bud.

"He's beautiful."

"Thank you," I said, looking at my wife.

"Barry will be pleased," she said, "having a baby brother—I wonder what he'll think . . . "

"Hush," I told her, knowing what *she* was thinking. "He won't envy his brother for being able to walk and talk as he grows. I don't think that Barry understands the differences. We've got Barry and we've got this one. Let's be happy on it as it stands."

"I'm glad for you," she said, clutching our son to her. "I really am glad for you."

"Yes," I answered, "I know you are. But I couldn't have done it on my own, so be glad for all of us."

3

The
Upper Window

ROBIN'S BABYHOOD and childhood familiarized him with Barry's condition from the start. He didn't ever question it; he accepted it. And as Robin grew into my life and became a main ingredient in it, it seemed to me that he served as a lubricant to bring Barry into the front of my life as well, so that gradually no distinction seemed to exist between the two, except in little impulses here and there—not exactly favoritism or preference; there *is* a word, but it eludes me. But because Robin was my son, Barry too became my son in every meaning and feeling of the sense surrounding the term.

Robin . . . we'd had no intentions of calling him "Robin," my wife and I. We'd decided to name him "Timothy." But my wife's brother said, "Robin's a nice name," and we agreed. Perhaps because I associated the name with the boyhood hero Robin Hood, the name conjured up images of a green and pastoral England, a spirit of adventure and of self-independence. The name seemed to fit; he'd got my Anglo-Saxon blood in him, light of eyes and fair of skin, in contrast with the darker Norman stock of his mother and Barry.

I don't really think Robin questioned Barry's condition until he was almost eight years old, when the first childhood innocence of life was floating away on the tide of increasing worldly experience. The fragile years. My wife and I had done our best to ensure that Robin's attitude towards Barry shouldn't grow hard and calloused. We showed him, gently I think, along the years, that his brother was representative of human chance illness; we made sure that stale familiarity didn't set in . . . but on the other hand we had to make sure that Robin didn't develop a personal guilt feeling in that he himself had full access to human faculties and facilities while Barry didn't. And again, we didn't want Robin to grow up feeling that he must assume fixed responsibility for Barry, based upon an imposed self-duty of kinship. We didn't want him to be bound to Barry because of blood relationship only. We wanted to make unnatural circumstances as natural as possible. We impressed upon him that Barry wasn't a "handicapped person," but that he was a *person* with handicaps.

I came to realize that very young children weren't put out by the physical handicaps of other children, or even of adults. In the early infant years they fail to make note of differences, because the infant years are the years of pure innocence. They haven't as yet been indoctrinated by the prejudices of adults long enough for the indoctrinations to make dents in their own personalities. Myself, as a boy, I knew a lad called "Saft Sammy." The adults called him "Saft" because he was "soft in the head," mentally retarded. We kids never thought of him as "saft"—he was older than us, chronologically, but mentally he belonged to our age group. Then, as we grew, we became aware of Sammy's "saftness" because adults said to us, "Don't get playing with that Sammy. He's saft in the head, he'll lead you into trouble." So eventually Sammy became "saft" to us also. A pity that the adults weren't enlightened enough to teach *us* how to keep "Saft Sammy" out of trouble, instead of telling us he'd get *us* into trouble.

When Robin was around eight years old I slowly became conscious of the fact that he wasn't fitting in, that he was on withdrawal course from the child social activities of his neighbohood. He became quiet, a loner, often listless. His work at school started to slip, he lost interest. And he lost personal courage or mayhap hadn't developed it.

From the upper window of the room in which I work at my typewriter I can see out into the lane. Often I looked out and saw that Robin was on the furthermost fringe of things with kids of his own age. They either ignored him completely or they noticed him only to push him around and bully him. I could see him forming attachments with smaller children, and in turn bullying them. Getting his own back, malforming emotionally. Looking down on him and them, I knew that Robin wasn't just passing through the normal scuffle stage of boyhood.

Something wrong was taking place inside him and overspilling. One of the lads in the group, bigger and slightly older than Robin, seemed to take particular pleasure in pushing him around; and Robin accepted the treatment, hangdog, almost fawning for favor.

"O Christ!" I thought, looking down on it all. "Robin's pushing his mind around in a wheelchair." Him down there. Lonely. And there was no way in which I could interfere. I couldn't go down to the boys and order them to accept my son. I had to give him something from me. Some invisible coin that would not diminish in the spending. I knew I'd got to give him some hard-core degree of self-confidence, no matter how painful it was going to turn out for somebody else.

I spent more time with him, talked and shared with him, trying to give him some clumsy home-spun encouragement.

"Look," I said, touching my face in several places, "a face full of scars. All from somebody's fists or boots. From when I was younger."

"They're not nice."

"I didn't ask for them. They just happened."

"How did you get them?"

"In defense of myself. By not letting certain people walk over me. By stopping them from hurting me even more—by protecting my own right to be *me*."

"Did they hurt?"

"Most of them. But it would have hurt me even

more, inside, if I hadn't made my stands. Look—I'm not saying you have to go out and earn scars. I'm not telling you to look for trouble and punch-ups. But I'm telling you this: walk away from trouble every time you can, if you walk away complete *inside* as well as outside. If walking away means losing your identity, your self-respect—if *that's* the price of walking away—then you must stand fast."

"But fighting hurts."

"Son, fighting does hurt. The pity is that sometimes we're forced to fight. I'm not asking you to turn yourself into a punching bag. I'm asking you to do it only the once. I'm asking you to go for that big boy next time he starts on you. I'm asking you to go for him hard and fast, to make his nose bloody, to make him cry. I want you to send him home running for his dad. If you do this, he'll leave you alone and the others will respect you. They'll know they can't push you around."

Worried eyes, blue-gray and serious, scared at the thought of fighting. Wanting to run away from the fight even before it was on the immediate agenda. But, in his boy-way, wanting the approval of his dad. And me, dad, hoping deeply that what I was telling him to do was the right thing. "Teacher says Jesus in the Bible says turn the other cheek," he whispered.

"Ask teacher to tell you the bit where Jesus drove the hypocrites out of the temple with his fists and a whip," I answered. "That bit's a bit more in keeping with the times."

My wife was angry with me that I should tell our son to go out and fight. "You're telling him to act like a barbarian."

"I'm telling him to act like a barbarian *now* so that he can be permitted to act civilized *afterwards*."

"There's enough trouble and violence in the world as it is," my wife said bitterly.

I snapped back at her, angry-protective perhaps.

"And most of *that* exists because people in the right of things won't swing a heavy enough fist to defend themselves. And to defend the values of life that are left to us."

Before the week was out I was sitting at my window, working at my typewriter, when I heard the children out in the lane. I looked down from the window, bird's eye view, and could see a ring of schoolboys. Inside the ring, two boys fighting, Robin and the bigger boy—I could see the flurry of fists, hear a wail of pain and protest. And the bigger boy came backing out of the ring, nose streaming with blood, eyes brimming with tears. And my son Robin standing there flushed and panting, a bit afraid of what he'd done. But *defiant* with it (that pleased me, the defiance). And I felt a perhaps permissible pride as the other boys crowded round him, slapping him on the back as if he were the Champion of the Ring ready to take on all challengers and newcomers. He shot into popularity that day and has remained there since, and up to

44

now I don't think he's raised his fists in violence again. If he has, he's never mentioned it to me.

It took me some time but eventually I got to the roots of his previous withdrawal and loneliness, his lack of friends; the period where he seemed to have no playmates of his own caliber. It wasn't easy, getting to the roots. I had to put bits and pieces together as I went along . . . but I found the trouble. Some boy in the playground had shouted out to him, "Your brother's a dummy."

Barry.

Barry sitting there at the downstairs window in his wheelchair, watching cars and people pass, watching the kids go to school. Jerking and gurgling overtures of friendship towards them . . . but to at least one of them he was a "dummy" and the contamination of the shouted, ignorant accusation spread across the playground to wound my young son with loneliness, and the feeling of being different. He was abnormal, subnormal, by association.

I kept the secret from my wife because the knowledge of it would have torn her to pieces. Alone, I thought about things—should I take Barry away from the window as the children passed by? Should we confine him to another room while Robin invited friends home? I asked myself these questions and felt the poison of self-anger boiling in my gut. Why not go the whole hog, I thought, and lock him in the cellar? Why not chain him to the wall and gag him in case he makes a strange noise? Why not give

45

him straw to sleep on and put the clock back to the days of Hogarth, of Newgate and Bedlam? And charge the public twopence apiece to come and see what I've got in captivity?

I took up my camera. I loaded with color-slide film and took pictures of Barry—happy, friendly pictures. In a few of the shots I showed a few of the lesser difficulties he had to contend with. I put camera emphasis upon his helplessness rather than the more grotesque aspects of his disabilities. Then I went to Robin's school and had a word with the headmaster; and he in his wisdom gathered the whole school into the darkened assembly hall while I projected slides onto a large screen and then talked simply about people with handicaps. I didn't mention Robin, or say that the person in the pictures was his brother. I kept it simple and uncomplicated. Then, at the end of it all, I asked the assembled—and attentive—children what *they* thought they could do to help such people. Silence. Thought. Then:

"Please, sir, we could knock on the lady's door and ask to take him out in his wheelchair."

"Please, sir, we could take him books and toys."

"Please, sir, we could go to the house and ask the lady if she wanted any errands run."

They argued and discussed among themselves the best things they could do; and having aroused in them some degree of insight I left them to work out for themselves how best to use it.

Robin formed good and close friendships from

then on; started to invite his favorite mates home for tea, sometimes to stay weekends and share his bedroom. And they came to accept Barry and treat his abnormalities with normality, and, who knows, in time they might influence their own parents and people in the neighborhood to adopt the same standards and attitudes. Not that their attitudes matter to us and Barry particularly now; but other Barrys will be born, to other people.

People in general aren't deliberately cruel in their indifference towards such as Barry—indeed, I sometimes wish they were, for cruelty of attitude requires effort and energy, means becoming aware and coming alive; indifference is a form of emotional death, inert, unproductive, nonvibrant, isolated. Apathy and indifference are the walls, the iron curtains that prevent self-harmony and harmony with others. The sick indifferences of the world start in ourselves, then infect our neighbors, our local streets and localities. It is from these small beginnings that apathy spreads out like cancer to pollute housing estates, villages, towns, countries, nations and continents.

4

Bruises

"How DID YOU FEEL when you first learned about Barry?" I asked my wife. "When they first told you what he'd grow to be like? Were you angry? Shocked? Frightened?"

"How would *you* have felt if they'd told you the same things applied to Robin?"

I thought back to the anxieties and depressions that had hit me when she was pregnant with my son. There was no answer, because my question was a meaningless one. There was no reality attached to it: how can someone make answer to a question that asks, "How did you feel when a part of you died?"

"The shock and the fear came later," she said to me. "At first I refused to believe—I thought they'd made a mistake. And then, when the truth did sink in, I felt as if all the world had died."

She'd had no idea for the first months of Barry's existence that there was anything wrong with him; she'd no insight, no warning, of the distress yet to come. She didn't suspect for a long time. Even when the first signs appeared.

"He became listless in his eating," she said, "and his neck muscles seemed to weaken. But his eyes were so intelligent, you know? They belied any indication that there was anything wrong with him."

But there must have been some subconscious suspicion in her mind. She took him to the child clinic every week, apparently seeking reassurances. "Pooh, pooh, mother," they said, "he's a perfectly healthy and normal baby."

"By the time he was eleven months old," she told me, "I realized that he *wasn't* normal. His thumbs had started to curve backwards . . . and his head leaned sideways, couldn't support itself. I insisted on seeing one of the doctors and he told me that Barry had an ear infection—that it would clear itself up, and all would be well."

She kept taking him to the clinic. She, little more than a girl herself, proud in motherhood, with just those tinges and taints of doubt at the edges.

"I was left alone in the clinic office for a few minutes," she said, "this one time . . . and I picked up Barry's file and read it. The file said that Barry was mentally subnormal and that he'd develop physical abnormalities. That's all I understood— there were official words I couldn't understand— and I thought it was a mistake. I thought Barry's file had got mixed up with another baby's."

She was silent for a while, looking in on her own thoughts and remembering. "Isn't it strange?" she said. "I felt this pity for the real mother, you know?

52

The mother of the baby whose information had been put in Barry's file by mistake. I felt this aching pity for her . . . but she didn't exist, because no mistake had been made on Barry's file. I was the mother I felt the pity for . . . but I didn't know it was me."

"Put Barry away," they eventually told her. The doctors told her when he was eleven months old, "put him away and forget about him, and have another."

Me as a boy in a farmyard near my home and the sow has farrowed and given out more piglets than she's got dugs for them to feed from, and the weak chap of the litter growing weaker and weaker. A runt from birth, and his siblings push him to one side as he and they squeal for the milk dugs.

"He winna mek it, Bill," the pig man says to the farm gaffer, and the gaffer shrugs, as indifferent as God.

"Put it down, then," he says, "and let the sow feed them as is fit." The pig man takes the piglet by its hind legs, it squealing and pleading to be allowed to live, and he dashes its head against a wall. The piglet is put down nastily while its community of brothers and sisters gurgle and grunt at the pleasurable udders.

"Put him away," the doctors said. To her, this mother, my wife. They did not look at her when they said it, they looked away; because if they'd looked at her they would have seen God-hope in her eyes, and they knew that God was gone away.

She didn't put him away. She took him away—

53

she took him away to her clean, sacred, secret places of motherhood; she took him away and kept him, and in the keeping relinquished most of her own life. Gave her own life as full extension of her son's.

I suppose when she took him home and didn't "put him away," "forget about him and have another," as the doctors advised, I suppose she hoped they were wrong. Made up her mind they were wrong. Why should she believe otherwise? Why should she disbelieve what her eyes told her? He was clean-limbed and perfectly formed. She doted upon a miniature of perfection which would soon show the development of gross imperfection. A dark-haired baby—brown eyes laughing out at the world and waving hands trying to grasp it—but gradually the power going from his hands, his body flopping like a rag doll's unless supported. I think she thought all this would pass away, that an error would be corrected, that his muscles would grow strong and he grow into straight manhood without impediment or blemish. I don't think, then, that she thought of her son being doomed to wheelchair imprisonment for all of his life and she a prisoner with him. Never able to follow her own whims, develop her own creativities, shape her own social life, always to be a servant-extension of him for every minute of every day of every year. Tied to him by fetters of responsibility as far as the casual outside world was concerned, but in her mind not tied by fetters but joined to him by love.

She wove, in those early days, dreams around her son. Long tender dreams which only mothers weave. But sometimes, despite her conscious will not to accept his subnormalities, the truth crept over the threshold of her frightened understanding; and she lay awake in the long darknesses of night cradling him in her arms, pillowing him to her breasts, sad and bewildered. Washing him with her tears. And sometimes, as time passed, the thoughts of self-inflicted death for herself and him trembled against her mind. Little more than a girl, she. Slim and dark and beautiful, with eyes rich in loveliness. She had hopes, sometimes, that her son would find normality, that something would click into place. It was mostly in the night hours that depressions dented her hope and left small bruises. . . . But she survived, and Barry survived, and twenty-seven years have passed since she first held him in her arms.

I recall more recent words spoken by my wife, at the time of the thalidomide shock, and they often burn at the back of my mind when I look at Barry. We'd seen, my wife and I, the news pictures of the thalidomide babies—brutally shocking. And then, as time went by and the babies grew and—to some brave extent—overcame some of their difficulties, my wife said to me, "I wish Barry had been born thalidomide. It would be a ninety-five percent improvement upon what he is."

I hope this God men talk of heard her say that, indeed I do.

I read, not so long ago, of a man who took his five-year-old mentally and physically handicapped son by car to hospital for a specialist check-up ... and they told him there would be no decrease in his son's handicaps, only increase. The man put his son back into the car and drove away with him. Drove him round country lanes, like lines of the poem which reads "... look your last on all things lovely ...," and he stopped the car by a river. He put his son into the river and let him drown and said in court, "I gave my son peace. I put him into the water and he floated away from me and my life went with him. ..." And more recently a member of the English aristocracy took the life of her badly handicapped child, "mercy-killed" it. Both she and the man who drowned his son—and how many others? —were sympathized with by the courts and let go free. The aristocrat, with her high standard of living, servants, private medical and nursing help constantly on hand to take from her the physical burden of caring—even she couldn't cope. It was too much for her, as it was for the father who drowned his son. So how do so many women like my wife cope? How do they manage physically, mentally, and emotionally? Not for three or five years, but for twenty-seven long, constant, droning years ... and some for longer than this.

Those parents who terminate the lives of their children in this way don't commit the act on the spur of the moment. The act of finalization isn't a sign that they are under strain but evidence that the breaking point of strain has been overstepped. The compassion and mercy of the courts is applauded when it lets strain-broken mothers and fathers "go free" . . . but what merit can there be in such applause or in the decision? Why wasn't breaking point averted, why weren't the pressures eased by State and Community, Church and Welfare? Why must so much social indifference make murderers of mothers and fathers whose basic desire is to love and preserve? The courts' mercy in every case such as these is an admission of the community's failure, and not its progress.

"Barry was such a beautiful baby," my wife said, the camera of her mind opening its shutter to pictures of the past. "I should have known such beauty couldn't last, that it had decay in the bud."

5

"Put off
thy shoes ..."

In relaxation he looks and is handsome. But when he's excited or agitated his face contorts and he jerks his body like a puppet-doll, whimpers and drools a bit.

"They should keep him away from people," I heard one self-contented lady say when Barry was whimpering his pleasure at a rare seaside trip. "They shouldn't let him spoil other people's holidays." I wasn't angry with the lady, not even contemptuous. What she'd muttered was of no importance. What *was* important was Barry enjoying himself.

He sits patiently in his wheelchair hour after hour, as if the world outside is a cinema screen with no continuation outside the frame of the screen itself. My wife and I are lucky that he's blessed with an even temper and seldom goes into tantrums of frustration. He sits there creaking and croaking his strange language.

Once, a passing drunk stood at the garden gate trying to talk with him. I watched from the inner shadows of the room, convulsed with laughter at the antics of the pair. Pleasure laughter, not grotesque. The drunk kept shouting slurred messages to Barry. Seeing him at the window strapped in a wheelchair, he probably thought he was a road accident victim or something. Barry gurgled and jerked at the stranger's attentions and the drunk took these as signs of encouragement that his messages of comradeship were getting through. Each time the drunk shouted a maudlin goodbye, Barry gurgled and gave a convulsive jerk, mouth wide open. And the drunk anchored back to position at the gate, thinking that the conversation was still in stride. Eventually somebody came along and "captured" the man and led him away, him shouting promises to come back soon for another interesting chat.

Sometimes I look at Barry and see that deep intelligence locked away inside him but trying to communicate with me. His eyes look at me wise as normality; and this frightens me, because I'd rather that there was no intelligence at all imprisoned inside his body. I try to identify with it and am afraid. What if I were strapped inside a space capsule, helpless but with my mind diamond-sharp, and launched into the unknown void to go on and on without any control over my speed, course, and direction? Without any control over the instruments of my vehicle—just housed inside it, helpless inside it, going on and on? Not even having the power of movement to self-destruct if I so wanted.

He had to stay in bed for a few days with a heavy cold and I looked at his empty wheelchair in the front room. Strange, looking at that wheelchair. It seemed to me that the wheelchair *was* Barry, like a workman's jacket—you've known the same sort of recognition; someone you know very well, and you see his jacket hanging on a peg and, despite the wearer's absence, the jacket *looks* like him. Each fold and crease, the way the garment hangs, the very shape it's molded itself into—that exists. As if the owner had passed his full identity into it, as if it were his skin rather than a dispensable item of clothing. Barry's wheelchair seemed like that. Not *of* him, but part of him. Strange. Not even a well-used motorcar takes on that sort of identity with its owner.

I sat in Barry's wheelchair. I pushed it to its usual position at the window and sat in it. Pretended I was Barry. For over a quarter of a century he has sat so. The chair is his home, its wheels are the full extent of his freedom. I sat in it and wondered how long I could sit there. I willed myself to be helpless. When my bottom grew sore through an hour of fixed immobility, I wouldn't move, because Barry couldn't move. He had to depend upon his mother or me to help him. A fly landed on my face and explored it, and I fought my hands from lifting to brush it away because Barry couldn't brush one away. A low-flying pigeon had splashed lime across one of the windowpanes, obscuring part of my vision into the garden. If I turned my neck a mere six inches I would be able to see past the obstruction and it wouldn't interfere with my vista. But Barry couldn't turn his head, so I didn't. I heard time passing inside my mind, unhurried time, monotonous time. I wouldn't let my hands reach for radio or television switches, because Barry's hands couldn't. Time was a funeral march inside and around me, slow-stepping, sonorous, meaningless and boring. Time was merely a bridge that had to be crossed, but in the crossing it grew longer and longer and led to nowhere. Time was an escalator but there was no way of knowing whether it was up or down, in or out. Time was time and there was too much of it. I closed my eyes and tried to daydream a bulk of it away, then opened my eyes because I remembered that I'd never seen Barry asleep in his chair. Always wide awake.

I couldn't see the room clock from where I was sitting. I could hear it, ticking away its tiny coughs but couldn't read the sweep of its face because that meant turning my head, and Barry couldn't turn *his* head. After a while I could hear the beat of my own heart, became conscious of it. Could hear the streams and oceans of blood pulsing through my own body, amplified by the shape of the chair around me, and my own inward-looking thoughts and concentrations. A cramp was in my left leg but I wouldn't reach down and massage it because Barry couldn't reach down and massage his. I thought a lot of time had passed. I thought many hours had gone by. I knew that the sun in the sky was a liar, that it had crossed more space than *that* ... I couldn't put up with it any longer, I had to get out of the chair and move about and feel my legs under me and scratch my face with my fingers, and go to the tap for a glass of water. I wanted to go to the toilet. I didn't want to sit in the chair and wet myself as Barry did, because he couldn't help it.

I looked at the clock. I'd been in the chair for two hours and thirty-six minutes. I thought I'd been in it hour after hour; but two hours and thirty-six minutes had been as long as I could endure. I left the chair, Barry's chair, and felt self-shame flooding through me, the shame of self for remembered self-pities, my past groveling pleas for help and understanding from my own self-made prisons of self-inflicted injuries, emotional and sometimes physical.

Only once have my wife and I rowed about Barry, some years ago when he'd grown into full manhood and needed shaving daily. Since I shave with steel and we daren't put a blade to him, we asked the local health authority to supply an electric shaver and also a food mixer, because his food has to be mixed to a pulp before he can swallow it. He can't chew, and a lump of meat or such catching in his throat might nigh on choke him. Both items were provided on request, the only material help we'd ever asked for. Then we decided to move and take Barry away from the concrete jungle of North London into the quietness of Hertfordshire, where he could get fresh air and see the countryside. When they learned that we were about to move, the authorities asked for the return of the razor and food mixer. And I said, "No!"

"You must return them to us and get replacements from your new county authorities," I was told.

"Return them," my wife said. "Give them back. Let's have no fuss—we can do without help that amounts to means-tested charity."

I was stubborn.

"I work out that *you've* saved the taxpayers around fifty thousand pounds by keeping Barry with you," I answered, "by not putting him into hospital or state care."

"Give them back."

"We keep them," I insisted. *"We're* reasonably articulate—but what about others less so but in the same position as us? We have to act for them as well."

We moved from the area, and within two months the previous authorities were on the doorstep demanding the return of "their" equipment.

"No," I said again, "this type of equipment should be provided on a national basis and not a local one."

They insisted.

"Give them *back,*" my wife said once more. "I will not have Barry cheapened."

"All right," I said, flaming mad, furnace raw with anger. "They can have them back—but they'll collect them from the editor of *The People* newspaper, where I'll deposit them and tell the editor why."

And they went away without their razor and mixer and never asked for them again.

Me, ripe with triumph.

She, my wife, scared and trembling with anger.

"Don't ever do anything like that again," she told me. "I will not have Barry made into a tug of war. I will not have him squabbled over like a dog with a bone." Her pride and independence is a currency beyond pricing, beyond estimating in value.

The aspect that moves me most, sears me with the deepest silent pity, is the attitude of my wife, her courage and devotion. A woman, like an unknown number of others, who has accepted the responsibility and burden without complaint and without self-pity; who *didn't* attempt to pass the burden on to state and taxpayer by "putting Barry away," as she was so often advised. And I worry because I know there must be a breaking point for women like her. Her energies feed on themselves, and I don't know what to do. More often than not I can only supply the muscle power, the manual labor of lifting and carrying Barry. Perhaps, sometimes, my services to him can be tainted with irritation or frustration. The imposed duties and obligations can sometimes intrude upon me, smother and irk me a bit, but *I* can often look at the clock for the freedom that my self-employment sometimes brings me. As I close the front door behind me I can leave the helplessness out of my orbit for a while. I have new things to do, new people to meet. There can be change in my life, distractions, some entertainment. But not for my wife. I try to puzzle it all out. I know that she still suffers heartache watching Barry struggle with his handicaps. Perhaps some husbands and wives come closer together in this sort of circumstance; perhaps others find an increasing strain put upon their relationship with each other; both may feel that their own inadequacies, real or imagined, are on show to the Outside World . . . a spiritual vitamin deficiency setting in, a shortage of neutral places wherein to repair their damaged emotional tissues.

My wife has had to forfeit so much of her own life, ambitions and privacies. There is no "clocking off" for her, no going on strike, no downing of tools, no pulling the switch to bring the machinery grinding to a halt. No Trades Union protection for such as my wife. No golden handshake and no pension or redundancy monies at the end of the treadmill for services rendered. No written contract of employment, no holidays with pay, no double-pay overtime, no perks and free coal and travel concessions, no "uncivilized working hours" remunerations. No pickets and banner-carrying demonstrations.

We have little social life together. The clock and Barry's needs are ever in her mind. Routines which

68

have no end, by which life is governed rather than measured.

During my military years as a regular serviceman there was a time limit to actual duty. So much time on active service, then home base and relaxation. Mothers like my wife have no such respites; life is one long-drawn battle, one mass of routine. We men have peak moments of sacrifice, over and done with in a fraction of time. Sometimes we strut smartly onto parade grounds to receive medals in velvet-lined boxes and live our small moments of glory forever afterwards, live and relive. Hand our valor down to our grandchildren, and adrenaline-spurted moments of valor, often with exaggerations of mystery attached. How cheap and petty so many of us can be . . . and which of us will remember women like my wife when they are dead and gone? I see no stained-glass windows to them, no memorials, no statues. But then, what form could a monument to love and patience take? Its essence could never be captured.

To know my wife is an experience that humbles. Outwardly calm and serene, she is a woman of great sensibility, charm, and intelligence. But the outer show of calmness and serenity is delicate and increasingly vulnerable. The long, hard and often lonely years have worn her to the very foundations, yet the foundations still hold. Sometimes attacks of migraine knock her sideways, exhausting her completely; but she won't give in to them. She fights

69

them away but I see the twin lines of pain furrowing her brow and something inside me wants to get up on its hind legs and throw tantrums and kick bits of life and the world to pieces, rip the cloth from clerics, blow the roofs off churches, and turn a machine gun against everything I don't understand.

Has my wife hoped? I think she has. Perhaps secretly, for that peace which must come with death, perhaps for cure and normalcy. Without Hope there is nothing. But Hope looks for miracles, and miracles are mirages that contain no substance. The one miracle that exists is the miracle of a mother's love. This remains, only this.

Barry's condition has deteriorated with the years. He weighs, now, about five and a half stone; and if we could straighten his limbs, he'd measure a reach of about five feet six. He's so helpless that he can't even turn himself in bed; one or the other of us has to do this for him when he whimpers from bed soreness. My wife measures five feet three inches. Times enough when she's been alone with him in the house and his bowels have opened unexpectedly, and she's struggled to stretch him out on sheets of newspaper and clean him up. And even when she can anticipate the opening of his bowels and we manage to get him to the toilet in time, she often has to sit alongside him for an hour or so, holding and supporting him, until he's finished.

Yet still, from the debris of the crippled body

that houses him, Barry shines through it all. Eyes quick to light with laughter, or sometimes silent tears of frustration. His eyes will always haunt me; the peepholes into his inner universe.

Lifting, carrying, bathing, hair washing, teeth cleaning, shaving, clipping his nails, toileting, unblocking his nostrils, changing his nappies—plodding tasks around which the whole of life must revolve and remain subordinate. I've constantly watched my wife involved in these tasks and have been moved beyond pity. Because in the final analysis I have always known that there could be no reward for her by way of recovery or improvement at the end of it all, only an increasing and perpetual geriatric-type deterioration. It's all been a case of Love's Labours Lost.

She is serene. I am not. I am conscious that in all our years together no neighbor has ever knocked on the door and said to me, "We'll Barry-sit while you take your wife out." She hasn't worn a dance dress in over sixteen years. In all our years together no member of the community has ever come to the door and asked my wife if she needs help with her son. Seven years we have lived in this house. The local vicar, who lives half a mile away, dropped by once. I told him that I wasn't a religious man, but that he would always be welcome at our house. To drop in for tea or coffee and chat to my wife about the neighborhood activities from which she is shut out. He came the once, five years ago, and came no more. But he preaches "Christian" love and compassion every Sunday from his safe little pulpit down the road—he and countless other simple, uninvolved people all over the world so ignorantly raising funds for church roofs instead of raising trust and hope in individual hearts, so very busy putting their "Christianity" onto pedestals instead of into circulation. But in the long run it doesn't matter, now. Neither my wife nor Barry has need of these, now; it is *they* who have need of her and him.

I draw the circle of my own love round them both like an amulet and will write the words from Exodus in large letters on the spot upon which they stand . . .

> And He said, "Draw not nigh hither: put off thy shoes from off thy feet, for the place whereon thou standest is holy ground."

6

"The windows
of the world"

"Why *don't* you put him away?" people have often asked us in the past, "so that he can be cared for and you be free?"

"No," I answer, "because if we did, what has taken my wife twenty-seven years to preserve and protect would be dead inside six months."

"Perhaps that would be for the best?"

"Perhaps. But he'll die when his time is due, and not for our convenience . . . we'll not let him die in torment of mind, silent and lonely, wondering why we've deserted him and left him to the casual efficiency of starched strangers in some dismal hospital ward."

"Perhaps he'd be happier with his own sort," comes the tentative suggestion.

Perhaps . . .

But we don't know, do we?

Because he can't tell us . . .

But he *can* tell us. He *has* told us.

The Welfare Worker came to see us, but my wife was out shopping, and I fixed matters up myself.

75

When my wife came home I had the exciting news ready for her.

"We can have a holiday," I told her, pleased as pleasure, "you, Robin and myself."

She was puzzled.

"What about Barry?"

"He's going to have a holiday too."

"Another caravan holiday?"

We'd done this before a long time ago—caravan holiday. We knew from experience that the likes of Barry weren't welcome at holiday guest houses and hotels. His strange noises and messy eating habits put other people off their enjoyments. I understood this. I didn't resent it. But caravan holidays never turned out to be holidays for my wife. Too cramped, too difficult in their fittings to manage Barry comfortably. And caravan holidays meant that my wife was more often than not tied to the stove. Holidays for Robin and me, yes, because we could wander abroad free as the wind on our own two feet. But most caravan sites were set in fields that made wheelchair-pushing of Barry almost impossible, so he'd sit outside the caravan in his chair, his mother with him. No family unity about such fragmented holidaying. Holidays in such circumstances were almost a dismal failure, so for years we'd taken none. Just stayed at home.

"There's a place in Hertfordshire," I told her, "where Barry can spend a fortnight's holiday—there's fully trained staff, lovely grounds—he'll be well taken care of while the three of us take a break."

We did just that, put Barry into the home for a fortnight and took ourselves off—the first time ever, my wife, Robin, and myself—and somehow we didn't enjoy it.

I'd seen my wife glancing at her wristwatch.

"It's Barry's lunch time," she'd say, as if to herself. Or, later in the evening, "It's Barry's bed time."

Barry was with us all the time. There seemed to be a sort of empty space among the three of us. Something vital was missing. I missed him. I'm not a sentimental man. I'm often accused of being hard; I know that I'm undemonstrative even with my wife and Robin, but that's the way I'm made. You don't necessarily lack love and affection merely because you don't put it on permanent show, with sign-boards marking where it is.

I'm not sentimental . . . but when I went to fetch Barry back home I shut myself in the staff lavatory and cried. I don't think I've every wept since I was a child, but I wept when I fetched Barry home. I looked at him sitting there in the ward and saw his face, and I turned on my heel and left that spot before my wife could see my own face, and I shut myself in the lavatory and I wept because the inner workshops of my emotions had suddenly been vandalized, smashed and crushed. I felt that a bruise had appeared inside my mind so big that people must see it.

After a bit I went back into the ward. Barry was sobbing his strange broken sounds, haunting wild sounds, like a snare-trapped animal in pain. His hands had found a strength and were clutching at his mother and holding her fast, and she was trying to free her hands to be able to cuddle him. And all the time the wild broken sounds coming from his mouth, the tears streaking down his face . . . tears and broken mouth-sounds were the only means of articulation available to him. And in the same ward with him, three dozen other victims of handicap; some terribly twisted and deformed, grotesque, as if they were members of some terrible circus freak show . . . a nightmare of humanity herded together, all together, so that the reality of the normal world outside seemed to recede and go away, as if it had never been. Strange sounds coming from so many strange throats, wheelchaired rows of strange throats making strange noises. The television set was switched on and for a wild insane moment I wanted to pick something up and hurl it at the screen, shatter it, and make the unreal people shining from it go away: lines of wheelchairs containing old men, young men, middle-aged men—*they* were the reality. Between them, they could clock up over a thousand years of imprisonment—there in that one room, over a thousand years of wheelchaired helplessness. I looked at my hands, looked at my feet. Strong and perfect. Ready to do my any bidding for good or for evil. I looked at the people lined up in the wheelchairs and hated myself for what I had been. For what I had done along the years, for the abuse I had inflicted upon the perfect machine which was my own body.

I carried Barry to the car, put him on the back seat, padded the cushions round him for comfort. His mother got in alongside him and held him firm for the ride home. I could see them both in my rear-view mirror. Barry's eyes were sunken, red-rimmed with weeping. His nostrils were flared wide, like a frightened pony's. Whimpers kept breaking from his throat, shaking his body in spastic tremors. My wife kept talking to him gently, soothing, calming, relaxing him from the fear that had held him for a fortnight, wiping the nightmare from his mind, the nightmare that we'd gone away from him forever. Crazily, lines from a Sassoon poem kept chanting away inside me: ". . . the windows of the world are blind with tears . . ."

I had to stop the car. I pulled at the hood-catch, got out.

"Got a loose plug," I said to my wife without looking at her. Under cover of the upraised hood I got myself under control, slammed the self-invented iron fist against the weepiness of my mind, made it stop. Got back into the car.

"It's the first and last time," I said. "We'll never do it again."

I could see her in the mirror, cuddling him to her.

"No," she said softly, so softly I almost couldn't hear her over the sound of the engine, "it's been no holiday for him. He's had two weeks of inner hell

79

. . . he thought we'd gone away and deserted him forever."

Later that evening I stepped into the bathroom and caught her in the act of making up her face in front of the mirror. I could see she'd been crying. I tried to jolly her out of it, bluff and brash from my own personal armor.

"It's all right now, lass," I said. "The lad's back home again—no need to cry on it."

There were deep pools of inward-looking pity in her eyes.

"It's not Barry," she said, "not now he's home again . . . it was that other wee chap in the ward . . . all doubled up and twisted, and blind and deaf as well . . . I was thinking of him."

I stood alone in the bathroom, looking at my own reflection. But I wouldn't, couldn't, meet my own eyes. I would have seen a degree of self-contempt in them. Contempt for the shallowness which was me measured against the vastness and profundity of the spirit of my wife. Not compassion only for her own son, but the pain and compassion stretching out to embrace other lonely and isolated strangers who had fleetingly touched our own personal orbits. I forced my eyes to meet my reflected eyes in the mirror, and saw and felt a sadness in them because I knew that my love and compassion for others could never be as deep and all-embracing as hers. And knowing this, I too felt that I was imprisoned with a personal handicap, that I too was inarticulate, that my mind was strapped into a wheelchair by safety belts, and that I had to wait for someone's love or compassion to move it about.

I have stood at the touchlines more often than not, the sidelines, watching my wife and her son. Over fifty years of devotion unite the two of them, the combined years of his age added to the same number she has given him in unselfish nursing. She, monument to patience; never complaining, or neglecting him, putting him first and foremost in all things, and always respecting him.

I used to think, in the early days, that a mother's love for her handicapped child was founded on sub-conscious guilt, in that she'd brought such accumu-lative helplessness into being; perhaps subconscious guilt for having wished the helplessness to have died at birth, perhaps guilt mixed with shame that the fruits of her body had been so sadly marred. But over long years of association with her I find no such guilt. Only love of a purity that surpasses my understanding. Sometimes in bed I lie awake and wonder about other women like her. I wonder at their difficulties, their extra problems. Wonder if they are tempted to creep into their crippled off-springs' bedrooms to put him or her out of existence with pillow over the face or a handful of sleeping tablets.

I'm often angry about things. My wife is never angry. Always calm and self-contained. She can put a remoteness around herself and Barry that nothing can touch, she can protect him with some invisible shield. I have no shield, only a sword.

Sometimes people come knocking at the door, strangers who are caught up in various cults of religious hysteria. Perhaps they see Barry at the window, or perhaps they hear about him from neighborhood mouths. Sometimes they come as "faith healers," or as self-appointed "witnesses" to some "Messiah." And they stand in the doorway like brush salesmen with one foot on the threshold, showing religious tracts and quoting from them, trying to gain admittance so's they can inject themselves with a main-line dose of their own uplifting fervor . . . hoping to hit the bingo jackpot of "Entrance to Heaven" through "Good Works." My wife is always polite with them, polite but firm. But mostly I am not. Sometimes I am rude and offensive, depending upon how much resistance they offer against my "Please go away." My attitude towards them mostly depends upon their insistence and persistence. One couple really got my fur bristling. They couldn't carry out a reasonable and rational conversation; their whole verbal exchange was made up of biblical quotes and had nothing to do with the real world around me. I felt a bit like a completely sober man trying to hold conversation with a drunk.

I grew impatient and let it show.

"Please go away," I said. "I don't believe in your god. Keep him and be happy with him, but I don't want to know."

Quote from this, quote from that; fervent talk about the Kingdom-to-come.

"Look at that lad," I said, pointing through the

side window at Barry in his wheelchair, "and then go away and think on why I won't believe in your god."

"Christ died for him," one of them answered, "to wash away his sins."

I laughed outright, almost with humor.

"What sins?" I wanted to know. "He's never been *capable* of committing any sins—he's more sinless than the Christ you're on about. Look, if you want to worship complete purity and state-of-grace and uncomplaining suffering, I'll let you kneel at Barry's wheelchair and worship *him*."

They were deeply concerned for my soul.

"God's hand is in that boy's condition," one said, looking in on Barry. "Whenever I see someone like that, I know that God is working in his mysterious ways."

"It's so bloody mysterious it's obscene," I answered, and closed the door in their faces. But they were Hounds of Heaven let off the leashes.

"We want to bring you to the Kingdom of Heaven," they called through the closed door. "We want to keep you from Hell."

Speed-of-light memories flashed through my mind of years gone by.

"I've been to hell," I answered back. "I've walked every inch of its paving slabs—have you?"

They popped some little tracts through the letter-box and went away.

"You were rude to them," my wife said.

I shrugged.

83

"They were rude to me," I replied, "by having the audacity to think I'd be interested in their claptrap."

She nodded thoughtfully.

"Yes," she said, "I think you're right—but *they* need help."

I marveled at her instinctive insight, her instinctive truths. Why don't they establish a Ministry of Compassion, I thought, and put you in charge of it?

There was a Western on TV. Which meant that my eyes would be glued to the screen for the next ninety minutes, which meant that my wife would bring supper and hot drinks on a tray for Robin and me . . . which means that she knows damned well that most men are kids again when the cowboys ride.

I settled Barry comfortably in his chair to watch with us. Just before the film started I sent Rob to his room to look through his put-away-toy box for a couple of "action-men" cowboys. He brought them down, dressed in full cowboy gear, with tiny pistols strapped into tiny holsters and stetsons on their heads. You could move the joints of the "action-men" and fix them in any stance or position. I tied lengths of black thread to the doll-cowboys, making sure that Barry didn't see what I was doing. I placed them on top of the TV set, bent their joints until they were part-crouched in the classic cowboy gunfight stances. Then I fetched one of my own pistols which decorate my workroom, an old American

Civil War cap-and-ball pistol. I primed the nipples with percussion blanks—they'd make a noise when fired but send out no missiles. I played around with the pistol in front of Barry so that his attention was caught by it. Then I sat down in my armchair, pistol in one hand and the ends of the black threads in the other.

The Western got under way and every now and then I'd raise my pistol at some villain on the screen, just to keep part of Barry's attention with me, and pretend to shoot at him. It got so that every time a certain "baddie" came into view, Barry looked at me and waited for me to "shoot" him. Came a certain moment in the film where a rifle sniper, was waiting in the rocks to pick off the "goodie." I raised my pistol, fired the primer-blank, and jerked one of the threads. One of the cowboys toppled from the top of the TV set. Barry's eyes were large pools of amazement. He looked at me with a mixture of laughter and admiration, and I raised the pistol for a second shot, fired, pulled the thread. The second cowboy hit the dust.

Then, all of a sudden, Barry was making these strange whinnying noises, his body heaving in the chair, breath gasping and rasping. His eyes were closed but tears streamed from under the lids. I grew scared and called for my wife.

"Come quick! Barry's having a fit!"

She came quickly, went to him, held his face between her cupped hands. Then she smiled.

85

"What did you do?" she asked. "He's only laughing—but I've never seen him ever laugh like it."

Relief eased my insides.

"We just shot a coupla guys off'n the TV set," I said in a John Wayne accent. I tried to put the pistol into his hand to help him squeeze off a primer round, just for the experience. But he flinched and winced away from the gun. I took the primer off the nipples and then closed his fingers round the butt. He accepted it, kept his fingers on it, although he couldn't lift the weight of it. A touch of bitterness tinged me.

"It's the noise, isn't it?" I said to him. "The bloody experts have been wrong all the time. You're not deaf. You heard the loud noise and didn't like it."

I switched the TV set off, put a Beethoven symphony onto the turntable of the record player. I placed one of the speakers on the tray of his wheelchair, a foot or so in front of him. I turned the volume up slowly, steadily. Nothing happened except that he kept looking with interest at the speaker. I pushed the volume up more, and his eyes started to flutter and his head winced as if he were trying to back away from the noise. I carefully softened the volume until I saw his face relax. I started to "conduct" the music, picked up Robin's school straightedge and waved it like a baton. After a bit I could see small fluttering movements coming from Barry's hands, small fluttering movements like fledgling birds stirring, little spastic jerky move-

86

ments as he tried to imitate me. He too was trying to conduct the music.

"I knew you weren't deaf," I said, putting the record away, "I always knew it. Oh, sod the bloody, bloody experts!"

Not long ago she called me to Barry's bed. She'd been giving him his morning sponge bath, running the electric shaver over his beard stubble. There was a deep frown between her eyes.

"Look," she said, pointing to Barry's groin. I could see a swelling just above the right testicle, a swelling about as large as a pigeon's egg. I put my fingers gently on the swelling, pressed lightly on it. He whimpered.

"What do you think?" she asked me. I felt at his sac. I could only feel one testicle inside it.

"Testicle's gone back through the aperture," I answered. "It's an undescended testicle."

"Will it come right?"

"We'll need to get the doctor in. If Barry's legs jerk together hard, he can crush the testicle and it will hurt . . . we could damage it just by lifting him."

The doctor came, examined the swelling, and agreed with me.

"Undescended testicle," he said. "It's a bit swollen and won't come back into the sac. I'll give him medicines to shrink it . . . best not to move him for a few days."

We kept him in bed, gave him the medicines.

But the swelling grew larger until it was the size of my clenched fist. The surface skin was bruise-colored from the pressures within. Barry whimpered and cried in the night from pain of it. The swelling was hard and hot. I called the doctor again. He was doubtful.

"We need a specialist opinion," he decided. "I'll get one in." Three days later the specialist too agreed that it was a swollen undescended testicle.

"But we'd best have him in hospital for X rays," he said. "We may have to operate." The ambulance came and fetched Barry away. My wife traveled with him. I followed behind in the car to bring her home again.

For the next few days the house seemed empty without him. His wheelchair in the corner of the room seemed sad with him not sitting in it. Then the hospital telephoned to say they wanted to operate, remove the testicle. Yes, I said, he has no need of it. We'd rather it were removed than have it happen again.

They operated.

"We'd best keep him in for a week," they told us.

"Can you manage him?" my wife asked. "He's very difficult unless you know what to do—difficult to feed."

"We can manage him. Don't worry."

But on our second visit the ward sister told us that they couldn't get Barry to take any food, so each morning early I drove my wife to the hospital and there she stayed all day to feed and nurse him.

88

I fetched her home around nine each evening, when all the patients were being settled down for sleep. Three days of it and the strain was beginning to show.

"You can't do it," I told my wife. "You can't keep it up—it's too much."

"I can manage," she said. "He's no trouble, I just want to get him well again."

Next day, when I took her to the hospital, I sought out the specialist in charge.

"It's too much for my wife," I told him. "She's spending all day here with Barry, then coming home and working in the house until midnight. Can't you bring Barry home again and have a nurse drop by to change his dressings?"

He agreed it would be for the best. But as the ambulance men were taking Barry out, he called me aside.

"I want to see you and your wife in a week's time," he said. "I shan't want to see Barry—just you and your wife."

I puzzled about it.

"The operation *was* a success, wasn't it?" I asked.

He seemed a bit vague.

"Oh yes, it was a successful operation. I just want a word with you and your wife next week."

She was troubled about it.

"Why want to see us?" she asked. "Why not Barry?"

After a while she seemed to relax.

"I think I know," she said. "Years ago they said

it was possible to operate on Barry, to cut certain tendons in his wrists and legs, that if the operation worked he'd have more use of his limbs. But I wouldn't accept it because they said there was less than a fifty-fifty chance of the operation doing any good—and if they failed Barry would be worse off than he is. So I turned it down. Probably things have improved in the medical field since then, and *that's* what he wants to talk with us about."

The week passed and on the morning we had to see the specialist I got myself ready, backed the car out of the driveway, then went back into the house to wait for my wife. She'd decided to leave Barry cuddled up in bed until we got back, with her mother to look in on him now and then. Her mother being eighty-four years old, we couldn't expect her to do much more. Then, as we were on the point of leaving the house, an ambulance pulled up outside, and the attendants came to the door and asked for Barry. "Barry isn't wanted," I said, surprised. "The doctor said he wanted to see my wife and me—he doesn't want Barry. We don't need the ambulance." One of the men glanced at his schedule sheet.

"It says so here," he replied. "Collect him for post-operation examination."

"We've got it mixed up," my wife said to me. "Of course they'll want to see how the operation is healing. We must have misunderstood what the doctor said."

The ambulance was waiting, the schedule sheet

had Barry's name on it . . . it seemed that we *had* got things mixed up.

"You stay at home," she said. "It doesn't need the two of us to go. The ambulance will bring Barry and me home again."

She quickly got him dressed and ready while I made tea in the kitchen for the attendants. Then they took Barry to the vehicle in his wheelchair, my wife with them, and drove away. I went upstairs to my typewriter and settled down to work.

About three hours later I heard a vehicle pull up outside and I looked from my window and saw the ambulance was back. The two men brought Barry to the house, my wife following behind. And I saw from my bird's-eye view that the whole essence of life and energy was drained from her, she seemed so shattered and broken. I watched this woman, this almost-stranger, coming up the driveway and I saw or I felt, I don't know which, a gray dull aura of sadness all around her, like a shadow blocking out the light of the sun.

I went downstairs and opened the door, and the ambulance men gave Barry into my care . . . they gave him to me gently and looked at me with some strange expressions of close friendship, and quietly they went away without speaking a word. And my wife slipped past me and went into the kitchen and I heard her filling the kettle at the sink, and I heard the gas jet hiss then plop its small explosion as flame ignited it. I placed Barry on the front-room sofa, his face looking up at mine, his dark brown eyes were smiling a greeting of return after the few hours of absence.

I went into the kitchen, where my wife was. She was putting out cups and saucers, pouring a measure of tea into the pot, waiting for the kettle to come to the boil. But she was mechanical in her actions, doing them but not doing them, being here but not being here. Her face was drawn, pale and tired. It was as if someone had switched a light bulb off inside her.

"Tell me," I said.

The kettle boiled and set up its wail and she mechanically reached out a hand to turn the jet down. She poured the scalding water into the pot.

"Cancer," she said, and her voice was flat and empty and without the luster and sparkle I knew so well; empty voice, sad and lonely . . . no music in it anymore.

Clenched mailed fist inside my mind. Slow motion everywhere, the world itself and all the broad invisible acres of Time gone into slow motion. "It was a mistake," she said, "the ambulance men coming. A mix-up. It was you and I they wanted to see after all, not Barry. They wanted to tell us that the lump they took from him was a cancer . . . it was all a mistake." I'd not been there. I'd let her go alone. I'd let her go and hadn't been there with her to take the first impact of shock, to soften it for her. The thought kept drumming in my brain—I'd not been with her to take the blow and ride it for her and to soften it a bit before it struck her.

I refused to believe it.

"It was a swollen testicle," I said, insisted to myself. "That's all it was."

"It was a cancer," she repeated, "malignant."

Malignant. What a terrible, shocking word; for the first time I considered the word itself. A dark, terrible word. Full of darkness and spite and malice, and overbearing power. An evil word, remorseless.

A week later we had to take him back to hospital for further tests. It was a different doctor; the one we'd been dealing with was away on holiday.

"Well, we'd best take a look at him," the new doctor said. We laid Barry out on the examination couch for him, peeled the plastic pants and then the nappy from him. The doctor probed at the scar tissue left by the operation.

"Healing very nicely," he said, "very nicely indeed. Right-oh, you can dress him again."

I was puzzled.

"What about the X ray?" I asked.

"X ray?"

"That's what we've brought him in for."

He glanced at his notes.

"Nothing about that here," he said. "The lad's fine enough—you can take him home."

I saw my wife's face lighting up, the lamp inside her lighting up again.

"You mean . . . there's nothing more wrong with him?"

"No, the operation was a success. It's healing nicely."

The light in my wife's face, in her eyes. Pleasure, relief, excitement bringing her towards the borders of hysteria. I slipped away. I went to the X-ray department.

"Look," I said. "Our lad was operated on for cancer. But a doctor out there says there's nothing wrong with him . . . that he's not booked in for X ray. But the doctor who did the operation, *he* saw my wife a week ago and said nothing could be done for Barry, that it was only a question of time and waiting . . . that the cancer would spread. . . ."

The X-ray specialist asked me for particulars. I gave them. She sifted and sorted through a stack of medical cards.

"Do you still live at Ware?" she asked.

I felt a sigh pass through every cell of my body. I felt as if my body were a vast forest and I could hear a great wind blowing through it.

"We've never lived in Ware," I said bitterly, "never in our lives."

"Oh Lord," she said, "we must have got the files mixed up."

The wind of the forest of myself stopped. I felt calm and composed, the anger gone away.

"You'd best get them sorted out properly then," I answered. "You'd best get in touch with somebody in Ware and let them know that he *hasn't* got cancer, before he kills himself under the strain of it all. Tell the man at Ware it's our lad who's got it, not him."

I went back into the hospital corridor. At the top end, caught in a shaft of sunlight, I could see Barry in his wheelchair with his mother cuddling over him . . . it was as if the sunlight were directed upwards from her and him, and not downwards upon them.

I went to them. Flat and brutal. Having to pierce and shatter the so-fragile globe of joy surrounding her.

"Stop being happy on it," I told her, and my voice wasn't mine; it was a hard stranger's.

"It's back to square one," I said. "There was a mix-up—Barry's got cancer."

"No," she said, smiling. "No."

"Yes," I insisted. I took her arm, twisted her towards me, made her look at me.

"Yes," I repeated.

I stood there and watched the light go from her again. Saw the darkness and sadness come creeping back. Watched the shadow pass back over the sun and stay there, with nothing left in the universe to move it out of the way.

Suddenly inside me the quietness of mind sharding and shattering so that I want to sink my fists into something, anything. I want to smash and savage and splinter and put my hands round the throat of chaos and choke it pleasurably. I want to blow up and out like a volcano. . . .

And then I don't.

All I want is to go home with my family, back to roots, back to some quiet decent sanity of safe familiar things.

"Let's go home," I said. "Let's take him home."

We pushed him down the long corridor to the ambulance outside.

"How long?" she asked me. "How soon?"

"I don't know. They don't know. It may be soon, it may drag on a bit. They said take each day at a time."

Her eyes were calm again. Calm in front of the sadness behind them.

"One day at a time," she said softly. "It seems all my life has been taken one at a time, every day of it. It's perhaps fair not to ask for more. Somebody once said that we all owe God a death."

We sat in the ambulance in silence for a while, then a thought struck me.

"You know," I said, "the doctor paid you a beautiful tribute."

"Tribute?"

"He said he was amazed Barry had lived so long ... he said people with Barry's condition usually died before they reached sixteen. He said Barry had only lived so long because of your love and caring for him."

She was silent so long I thought she hadn't heard me.

"What a strange thing to say," she said at last, more to herself than to me. "What an almost terrible thing to say. Of course I love him . . . he's my son."

I cleared my throat.

I knew my voice was going to come out gruff, self-conscious.

"I want you to know," I said "—and I wish Barry could know—I want you to know that I owe you so much, both of you. I have to tell you. I might go through all of my life and never say it again. But I want you to know."

"Shropshire Lad," she murmured. "I know . . . you don't have to tell us. We know."

I felt suddenly shy as a schoolboy.

"Thanks anyway," I said. "Just . . . thanks."

7

Footprints

A FEW DAYS after Barry came home from hospital, it snowed. A freak storm of snow . . . mild spring suddenly went away, leaving a gray dull sky and coldness of earth, cold whiteness. But here and there in the garden a gleam of yellow startled through the whiteness where the daffodils bloomed. The green leaves stood out like sharp scars, and the yellow flowers gleamed bravely, polished by the saps of spring. And here and there red flower-blooms showed bright as wounds, splashes of blood.

I called for my young son and at the magic word "Snow" the sleepiness left him and excitement washed his mind. He was rinsed and dressed and at the breakfast table before the kettle had boiled. His blue-gray eyes filled with a delighted wonder as he stared out at the unexpected vision of a white-clad world. His twelfth such vision—few enough, yet, to fill him with magic wonder. It was my forty-ninth such vision—many enough to erase the magic and wonder, leaving impatience in their place. Impatience for spring to come into its own again and stretch into a long green summer. Thirteen-year-old boys see snow as a swift carpet to race sleds across,

as substance for sculpturing snowballs and snow-
men, as nature's tinsel and cotton-wool, with which
she decorates trees and hedgerows, fields and roof-
tops. Middle-aged men like me see snow as tomorrow's slush and nuisance, see it as stiff-bristled
brooms with which to scrub driveways and paths,
and Wellington boots stored in little cupboards
under the stairs.

I put my target rifle into the boot of the car,
camera bag on the back seat.

"Will you come, and we'll take Barry?" I asked
my wife.

"You and Rob go," she answered. "He doesn't get
much of you to himself—you and he go."

"I thought the run might buck you and Barry
up a bit."

"He's sleeping—let him sleep."

The two of us, my young son and I, drove into
country lanes, which seemed strangely narrow
now that snow-heavy trees hemmed them in. Snow
purred and slushed beneath our wheels. The car's
interior was solid with heat, making the cold white
world outside seem as if it belonged to a television
screen, scenes passing by. I stopped the car in an
open space of flanking woodlands, took up my
camera and we got out. The coldness snatched at
us. I asked my son to walk towards the trees, turn
and come towards me with his duffle coat unbut-
toned. The bright scarlet of his polo-necked jersey
was an eye-wincing stab of color in the pentaprism
of my camera. The backdrop of trees, white-

shrouded and blue-misted, made him seem small and forlorn. So young and fragile. I took shot after shot of him to store against my future years, when his childhood would slip away from me forever.

We walked deep into the woods, the silent woods disturbed from a white sleep by our footsteps crunching by. Behind us our footprints stood out dark and sharp. Mine large, his smaller. They stood out dark and sharp, footprints which would lead to a beginning if we retraced them; but up ahead, nothing which would lead to an end. Only a blankness, untouched. No footprints leading to, only from.

A strange feeling, no doubt brought on by the white silence, gripped me. I was looking down on a wide vast domain of snow-covered time. I could see my footprints imprinting into the snow, advancing, and my son's advancing with mine. And then, after certain time and distance, my footprints stopped and his went on alone and grew to manhood as they traveled. An inextinguishable anguish wrenched my gut and I clutched the boy to me. "As long as you don't have wheelchair tracks mixed up with your footsteps," I said aloud, thinking of Barry back home; thinking of the children my son would one day have, wondering if there was already an imperfection inherited into his own genes waiting to be passed on.

He was puzzled.

"What's the matter, Dad?"

I was conscious of still holding him.

"I slipped," I said. "Thanks for saving me."

He was wiser.

"You were thinking of Barry," he said, "when you talked about the wheelchair."

"Aye," I answered, "I was a bit."

We pushed deeper into the woods and the sun came out to make searchlight pathways through the glooms. Backlit, the snow seemed suddenly like tiny glass beads individually heaped on and around each other, each with its own center rainbow of light. The sun, seen through the branches, was more like a many-pointed star on a Christmas card than our familiar sun of globe-shape. There was a magic in the woods which wafted pollen scents of rare memories of my own boyhood, when I'd sometimes walked out with my own dad. Misty years ago. His footsteps had stopped so long ago, leaving mine to go on until they were joined by those of this, my son Robin.

His mind, sensitive to mine, was uneasy. I tried to dispel his mood and mine, to make it a time of sharing with him, not wanting the blackness inside me to frown against him.

"Rabbit tracks," I told him, pointing, "just there."

He examined them dubiously.

"How do you know it's a rabbit? It could be a badger or anything."

"Look at the front pad marks," I said, "small and deep. Now look at the back ones—long and flattish. Short front legs, long back ones. It's a rabbit, a hopper."

"It could be a hare."

"The strides would be longer, further apart. A hare leaps, a rabbit hops—unless it's raised by a gun or a dog, and then it scuds."

"What's 'scuds'?"

"Means it goes like the clappers of hell—same type of spoor, but he *moves*. This one was dawdling, taking his time." I put my hand down and felt a pile of rabbit-pills.

"Still warm," I said. "He's not long gone this way." We followed the tracks, noting the places in the woods where the rabbit had scraped snow from tree roots and shrubs in search of food. I heard wood pigeons cooing and roaring. More rabbit tracks crossed and crisscrossed, with several droppings of pills. I hesitated.

"There's quite a few around," I said. "We'd best go back to the car."

"What for?"

"Leave the camera and fetch the rifle."

Gray eyes on mine.

"What do you want the rifle for?"

"Get a rabbit for the pot. Maybe two or three. They're good eating, are rabbits."

Gray eyes hard.

"No!"

Surprise inside me, tinged with anger.

"Don't be silly. Rabbits are for eating."

"It's cruel."

"Is it cruel if a fox gets one?"

"That's different."

"Is it cruel when you sit down to a dinner of lamb chops or steak or pork? Somebody had to kill the lamb or the bullock or the pig—"

"That's *different*."

A hardness inside me, hardness for his sake, for his protection.

"Steaks and chops don't grow on trees, chap," I told him. "They're born, bred and slaughtered— and mayhap not killed as quick and clean as I'd drop a rabbit with a .22."

His mouth was hard with resistance; a boy from a protected world where meat is ready-grown inside plastic wrappers under the roofs of supermarkets. Boy-innocent, knowing nothing of death's urgency, living inside a closed world he wants to go on for ever and ever. How tell him that death is the tormenting shadow of everything that lives, waiting to step into the substance? How tell him that my footsteps will one day cease to advance with his?

I collected twigs and small branches.

"See, like this," I said, and took my jackknife from my pocket. I shaved thin slivers from a branch, fine as rice paper, a handful of them. I scooped away a small circle of snow, placed the slivers on the cleared ground, built a pyramid of twigs and branches over them. I placed the smallest and driest twigs next to the slivers. I was trying to win my son to me with remembrances of my own distant woodsman's magic, taught to me by men of my boyhood, when my father had poached to put food on our

106

table, during the Great Depression. My own son had always known me as a townsman, and I wanted to show him deeper than that.

"See," I said, "supposing your matches were wet?" I pushed a red-tipped match into the snow, moistened it with my mouth to make it wetter.

"It won't strike now," he said, curious.

"Ah," I answered, and pushed the wet match into my hair, against my scalp. After a couple of minutes the match was dry again. I lit it, put it to the wood slivers. They glowed with tiny fire-life, tiny flames. Then the twigs flared, and soon the small branches.

He laughed at the simplicity of it. We squatted round the small fire, cupped our hands over its warmth.

"Now," I said, "imagine we're in the middle of Alaska—we've got fire and we've got water because we can melt snow. So what do we do about food?"

He avoided my eyes.

"We go hunting?" he asked at last, small-voiced.

"We do," I answered, "or we die from hunger. We can hunt rabbit, elk, bear, geese—anything. Or we die."

He thought about it.

"We're not *in* Alaska," he said. "We can buy food in the shops. We don't have to kill anything."

I sighed.

"If there's a war when you grow up," I said, "you'll shoot men."

"That's different."

I was angry.

"It's always different when you want it to be. You're old enough to *know* that life isn't all pretty pictures. In life, in nature, it's survival of the fittest. Only the fittest survive in nature, except man. Man's the only animal who lets the unfit survive."

He'd walked from me. His voice came back as lonely as the snowscape.

"I don't want to know. I don't have to know."

I doused the fire with snow, followed him back to the car. I didn't speak to him. I took the gun from the boot, walked back into the woods, knowing that he was following me. I sighted up on a wood pigeon, fired, and killed it. He ran to it. While he was looking down on it I sighted up and shot another.

"You did it again," he whispered, white-faced. "You did it again." I ignored him, picked up the plump birds and put them into the car boot for plucking and cooking.

He was silent beside me in the car as I started the engine. I tried to make him understand.

"Everything has life," I said, "even the corn which makes the bread we eat had life. Every time we eat, we take life. Fish, fowl, animal—it all had life before we took it away. We just have to content ourselves with the loose thought that only human life is sacred and special, and all other life is a means to preserving that life. Every time we walk, take a stride, we kill life . . . insects, microbes . . . it's all life and taking of life."

After a bit he said, "Barry's ill, isn't he? He's not well?"

"No. He's not well."

"Is he going to get better?"

I failed the question, concentrated on the driving. The sun was now high and strong, melting the freak snow swiftly. The roads were wet with water. Only the fields were keeping thin white mantles for a bit longer, drawn over them like bedsheets.

"I'm out of pills for Barry," my wife said when I went indoors. "I miscalculated."

I drove to the surgery, collected a prescription, took it to the chemist's shop, and got the pills. I got back into the car and drove away—then my heart lurched sickeningly as, against my inside mirror, I saw a glimpse of face bob up from the back seat. I braked hard, swerved curbside, stopped and turned. My young son Robin there on the seat where he'd been hiding. I swore at him.

"Christ!" I bellowed. "What the bloody hell are you playing at?"

His face was frightened at the thunder in my voice inside the enclosed car.

"I walked to the doctor's to meet you," he said, "The car was outside. It wasn't locked so I got inside."

"You hid under Barry's blanket," I raved. "Bloody young fool! I could've had a heart attack, I could've thought it was a mugger—anything!" I saw the fear in his face and forced myself to relax into calmness.

"Okay," I said. "Forget it. Climb in beside me."
He came into the passenger seat.

"I was worried," he said. "You acted strange in
the woods . . . and then you went to the doctor's. I
thought you were ill—what did you go for?"

"H'mm?"

"Is something the matter with you?"

"No, I went for Barry."

Silence. Then, "Is he very ill, Dad?"

"Yes."

"Mom said she wants him to die before she does,
or before you. What does she mean?"

"She'd mean Barry would pine without us—he'd
be sad if we weren't here. He loves us."

"I love him as well."

"I know you do. We love each other, all of us.
We're a family—the most precious unit on earth."

"When will he die?"

"I don't know . . . it may be quick, it may be
long."

Left foot thrusting the clutch down, left hand
shifting the gearstick, right foot blipping the
throttle. Both hands to the wheel, steer the familiar
corners—blossoms out on this corner, yellow and
green and rich with thrusting life. All snow gone
away now, and a sky so blue as to seem impossible.

He spoke quickly to make my words go away,
spoke quick and high.

"Look," he said. "Jimmy Large—he's in my class
at school."

I pipped my horn for Jimmy Large on my son's behalf. They waved to each other like lovers.

"See," he said, "Mrs. Watt's dog outside the shop waiting for her . . ."

"Dad," he said, "why do you like Stafford bull terriers . . . ?"

"Dad," he asked, "when shall we have a new car . . . ?"

"Dad . . ." he said.

I stopped the car inside the driveway. We sat looking through the windscreen as if we were still traveling. All the snow was gone away now, every crystal of it. The squirrels were out and about in the trees, showing off to their own self-importance and self-confidence. The rich smell of spring, the secret-sacred Woman, was filling the world. Blue tits were feeding from the gauze bag of bacon rind my wife had put out for them. I watched the tits and wished one of them would go to Barry's window and flap wings full of color, specially for him, and talk to him in Hiawatha language.

"Son," I said to his blue-gray eyes, my young son sweet of face and clean of limb, "son, there are sad days ahead . . ."

"Yes," he said, holding my eyes with his as if he expected some magic from me, some magic to take the nastiness away, like a dad's hands brushing the nightmares from the brow of a sleeping child.

"You know, don't you . . . ?" I asked him.

He put his hands over his ears and rocked his

body sideways and sideways, moaning strange and sad. I reached out to him and stilled him, willing quietness from my hands into him. And he became quiet.

"Yes," he said, "I know."

His boy-small hand touched mine on the steering wheel.

Later my wife said to me: "Go to Robin. He's in the garden shed, crying." I went to the shed. I could hear him weeping. As if his heart would break. Him in there in the dark and gloom of a shed filled with car bits, lawn mowers, bicycles, house paint, stepladders and household "maybe-we'll-need-its." Seated on an upturned bucket, eyes blurred with tears.

"Tell me," I said, "which part of it worries you most?"

"All of it," he whispered. "Why must Barry die?"

"We must all die."

"To go to God?"

"I don't know."

"You don't believe in God. I've heard you say so."

"Do you believe in God."

"I—think so."

"Then why let my unbelief trespass upon your belief, son?"

"I don't understand."

"If every son did as his father did, or believed as he did . . . man would still be at the cave level."

"I don't understand."

"It doesn't matter."

"I want it to matter."

I thought on it, dug for answers. There were none.

"Rob," I said, "I could fob you off. I could tell you that you're not old enough to understand . . . but what I'd really mean is that *I* don't understand."

I sat by my urgent frightened son there in the dark and smelly shed, with thin lances of sunlight poking in at the narrow window. Birds were singing. Spring-songs, courting the sunlight and each other. I thought of the dead pigeons and wondered if the shock of shooting them had been too swift and sudden for a bemused boy . . . but there was a hardness in life that he had to meet, had to accept. He'd fallen asleep against me, tight in my arms. I sat on with him, feeling the warmth of his body pass into mine. In some strange way, holding my son, I felt that in my nursing arms I held myself.

8

"Do not go gentle ..."

His FINGERS LONG and white and slim, the nails beautiful and elegant. Neatly trimmed and manicured, gentle with helplessness. Two of his fingernails shining like wax polish where my wife has buffed them, giving them a pearl-luster. I watched her do it, knowing that it was contact with his flesh she was seeking, but trying to give some purpose to the contact. I look down on her as she looks down on her son, loving him with her looks, wanting to die in his stead. Her eyes told that—that she would die for him because she had lived for him a long twenty-seven years. My face a neutral mask hiding a critical mass of thoughts ever boiling and exploding, ripping me to pieces inside.

"Look at his hands," she said to me. "They've never hurt a living thing. . . . All they've ever reached out for is Trust. . . . Why?"

But I fail the question, I have no answers except clichés. I fail the heartbreak in her voice, I fail to mend the broken chaos in her eyes. I turn to the window to look out at the new spring's promise, at the green flush spreading on trees and hedgerows. Red blooms stain the air like so many robins' throats. Beyond the lawn the daffodils still dawdle, yellow heads reaching for the sun. The squirrels are out and about and they amaze me. Not afraid of height, they trapeze from branch to bough as if confident that a safety net awaits to catch them. But a noise from an earthbound human in the lane sends them leaping across chasms of space in alarm, putting risk where none should exist. Two pigeons, a courting couple, perch on a branch that overhangs the driveway. They splatter droppings of lime where people must walk and I move without thinking to fetch the rifle. Then stop and don't go for it. I stand at the window and give my mental permission for the courting pigeons to splatter as much as they want . . . who am I to snuff their lives out?

My book near the lad's bed, my book of Dylan Thomas. Mr. Heartbreak-Dylan Thomas, you Welsh thiever of the fabric of men's minds—why do you haunt with your "Do not go gentle into that good night . . . Rage, rage against the dying of the light . . ."? Too many times in my life you have raged that rage against me but never as keenly as now. If I shoot one of the pigeons, will the other come raging against me to revenge it? Will my wife's son there on the bed—will he rage against the fading of his light? Is he raging now in the deep silent reaches of self? Will you or someone or anyone tell me where God lives so that I may go to him and rage against him? My thoughts are fierce sparks from a loud anvil inside my mind.

Her dark eyes on mine, clear of eye-tears, deep with soul pain. "Give me hope," the eyes ask me, "give me hope."

"God will love him," I hear my lying lips say, speaking empty words, words printed in Letraset: words which have form and shape and surface communication, but no meaning in themselves.

He has messed himself. I can smell it. We clean and change him . . . she has been doing this for twenty-seven years, my wife. Simple arithmetic tells me she's changed over thirty thousand nappies for him—each one has to be slightly more than two feet long . . . she's changed over twelve miles of nappies for her son.

I put my left arm under the crook of his legs, lift his buttocks clear of the bed. My right hand unbuttons the waistband and flies of his trousers, peels the garment down to his ankles. She slips sheets of newspaper under him to catch the mess and stains as we take the plastic cover-pants from him, then the fiber nappy filled with body waste. I keep him fixed and still so that he can't spread the mess, while she takes the soiled rubbish and puts it inside a small disposal bag and seals the end. Together, we sponge and wash him clean. His pubic hairs sprout strong again, his penis increases a slight length as the warm water invigorates it. I look at his penis and my mind is poisoned with rage again: this child-man rotting away when he should be in the full flush of proud fatherhood.

I suddenly want to hold him, cradle him in my arms, kiss and love him. I want to protect him from death, the last goodnight. I want to rage against the fading of his light, no matter it has always been a half-light. I want to hold him, comrade him, brother and befriend him . . . but if I do any of this my reserves will burn away and my wife will burn away too. Keep it calm, keep it simple, keep it emotionally uncluttered.

We talcum his buttocks and groin. A safe smell, a sweet, family, Woolworth's smell. His dark-haired head on the pillow. As it turns I see a glimpse here and there and a ghost of his mother, a sigh and a promise of her, a quickened likeness that appears and is gone. From the corner of my eye I watch his mother—so beautiful when I met her, so lovely, so full of pure life. Faded now and tired, a tired monument to sacrifice.

We sit quietly in the front room while Barry sleeps. The clock ticks like a faraway woodsman hacking down trees. We hold a silence between us which looks for a bridge to get across, we grope for a lamp to see by.

Who am I, sitting here and, by listening to silence, trespassing upon it? . . . Who am I in contrast to this woman, this mother, this sacrifice who waits for her son to die: who has so achingly often wished her son may die before she does, to die before she is too old and tired to look after him anymore? To die and be safe.

But not this way. Not at the end of a treadmill of absolute helplessness to die through rotting inside.

She sits, part tired, part lovely, in the light and shadows spilled softly from a single standard lamp. The clock ticks its urgent message, metallic heart grinding time away. The dog Candy sobs in sleep from the hearthrug, chasing a rabbit through a dream of fields. A sigh of wind troubles at a loose window sash, like a faint ghost seeking warmth and companionship. I see tears like seed pearls stroking my wife's cheeks, slim pale fingers, transparent rivulets.

"It was a lonely dream," she says, murmurs, "last night. I dreamed Barry was dead and done with, and I'd got used to it. I'd got over it . . . it was all finished. But in my dream I had to go to this place . . . a medical place, and there were these doctors. You were there, but it wasn't you . . . I knew it was you, but you were different . . . and they had this baby with them. It was, oh, such a beautiful baby . . . and I wanted it for my own. And they said I could have it . . . and one of the doctors smeared stick-stuff over the baby's face. And the baby tried to wipe it off with its tiny hands but couldn't . . . and the doctor said, 'There, I knew it was mentally retarded.' "

The tears down her face traveled twenty-seven years.

"Hush," I said, gruff as gruffness, "it was only a dream . . . only a dream."

Upstairs, our other son. Young and green and

straight in limb and sharp in mind . . . no litter-runt, he.

"Will he hurt?" she asked me, tired in the lamp-light. "When the time comes for Barry, will he have pain?"

"He'll have no pain," I answered. "The doctors said there'd be no pain. They'll drug him when it's needed . . . then, one time, they'll increase the dose." ("And if they don't," I said to my thoughts, "I will do it myself. Swift and clean and final.")

"His mind will ride out on pretty pictures," I said. "His mind will go out from his body and it will be happy, because it won't come back."

I went into the kitchen, made cocoa. Hesitated, then melted a sleeping tablet into her cup.

"Come to bed," I said. "I promise, they'll be kinder dreams tonight."

She went into fast sleep. I lay staring at moon-light through the window, listening to owl calls . . . mournful as fogbound ships. She whimpered in sleep and I felt uneasy about the sleeping tablet I'd given her. What if a dream were holding her and wouldn't let go? What if I'd switched her body off but not her mind; she sleeping there, trying to waken from a dark forest of nightmare but not able to?

I got out of bed and went to Barry. He was grind-ing his teeth as if he wanted to turn them into powder. I untangled the twists of his limbs, turned him onto his opposite side, worked his shoulders forward so that his arms were free and his body weight wouldn't cause cramps or numbness. I looked down on him and thought how easy it would be to take up the pillow and put it over his face, bear down on him. A few moments and it would all be over, and him free at last. But he came awake and looked at me, and his eyes were dark and bright as knowledge. His tongue, curving across his lips, told me he was thirsty. I spooned water into his mouth and his throat gurgled on the swallowing of it. I tucked the bedclothes around him and he made sounds of gratitude, little broken sounds struggling inside him, looking for a doorway to come through. Puppet creaks and noises. His body was thin as neglect, the bones of him standing sharp. No amount of feeding and coddling him could help him put weight on. I marveled that such a body could have kept the flame of life burning for so long and had contempt for Creation that life was given in the first place. Kind moonlight painted his face. A boy-face, with a man's stubble of beard thrusting its roots towards morning. Strong dark hair, wiry and curly. Brow smooth as peace. His mouth in repose was firm but gentle, with uplifts of humor at the corners. Stale bed-smell to him . . .

God and Christ didn't say, "Suffer little children to come unto me"; they said, "Let little children suffer." As this one has suffered for so many long droning years.

When this lad was born I was twenty-two years

old, quick with young manhood, eager as the blood which drove me along, reckless and ruthless as youth's uncertainty. When I was so, this lad could never be so. When he was twenty-two, he'd spent all those years locked inside a prison of useless flesh; no external signs really indicated whether the computer of his mind was fully at work. I hope it was not. Because if it was, if it has been, then he has been a castaway marooned in utter isolation on a tiny strip of land poking up from a dark deep sea, deep and dreadful and lonely. I stand looking down on him, wishing for quick, not lingering, death to wipe him clean, to blow his candle flame out.

I look in on our young son. His thirteen years of age are fast asleep. He too has uplifts of good humor at the corners of his mouth. Face flushed with the richness of good sleep . . . head on pillow, beside him his steadfast friend from babyhood, the teddy bear. Old and tattered, with one glass eye missing; here and there patches of bare fabric lost to loving cuddles. Ears ragged and tattered, eroded by nighttime whisperings.

In the corner of the room, his fishing rods and punching ball. Laid out on a chair, his football kit. On his night table, a cap pistol to keep away the dangers of night imagination. Spread around his bedroom are the contranklements of growing up . . . but in the bed with him, warm and secure as he is, a teddy bear that still keeps him in childhood pastures.

How can I tell him that there is no permanence in life, only in death?

I stand at the window watching the moon melt on the darkness, and the night wind tugs at the world like a sad, sad music.

9

The
Secret Garden

IF ROBIN HADN'T BEEN BORN, perhaps I would never have learned how to love Barry; I may have increasingly hated him, I don't know. And now, perhaps I love Robin more than I love Barry . . . but there are different layers of love, although equal.

Robin is a boy who runs to me, happy in the coming, joyful in the union of father and son. Barry I have to go to, lean over, make comfortable, lift and carry. I can enter into Robin's life and share it, but cannot enter into Barry's, only guess at its inner dimensions and wonder what goes on inside his mind. I wonder if he's lonely in there, so cut off, so amputated. An unpleasant death is filling him up slowly inside, invading him cell by cell . . . a Black Hole in his inner universe is eating him up. Sometimes in his eyes I see that dark aliveness staring out at me, an equal intelligence . . . and I find myself waiting for him to speak. The moment becomes electric with the expectancy that he will speak. Our eyes hold and lock to each other and I see that deep utter intelligence looking out at me. And then it fades and is gone, and the eyes of him look in on self alone.

I have learned rich things from Barry. When I

am an old man I shall look back on the memory of him and know then that the richness of his influence upon my thinking, upon my compassion and understanding, was of the very stuff that stars are made of. Not glittering baubles hung in the night sky to light the way home, but complexities of design and construction beyond all earthbound comprehension. He has been, to me, a solemn music made up of many melodies, some sad, but equally some gay and happy. I think above all I will respect, in the small core of my center-being, the trust and affection he has had for me. I will remember, always, the gladness of my coming lighting up his eyes. His eyes I shall remember, talking to me. Not of my blood, Barry, but of my center-being. Deep of it, because he has added dimensions to it.

This morning I stood behind his wheelchair in the downstairs room, looking out of the window at what the spring sunlight painted. He was locked in on his own thoughts. I stood behind his chair and tried to see what he could see. I mentally locked my feet against the floor so that I was helplessly fixed to a single position dependent on someone to move me . . . it seemed years since I'd sat in his chair that day and endured two hours and thirty-six minutes of nothingness and self-imposed helplessness. . . . I again tried to see what he could see, and it was a small enough world. His wasted neck muscles gave him no more than thirty degrees of head turn; they narrowed his vision to almost frontal. I tried to imagine how many incompleted scenes and dramas passed his eyes each day as he sat in his wheelchair. He could see people and events pass in front of his eyes but couldn't turn his eyes to follow them to some sort of conclusion. A dog ran past us but Barry couldn't turn his head and see it join its owner, as I could. The bird which carved the sky in front of us, he could not see where it landed on the tree beyond the range of his head-turn vision. Housewives with shopping bags passed up and down the lane, passing left to right across his vision as they went to the shops, or right to left when they came home again. He knew many of them by sight through long hours spent at the window and gurgled greetings which they couldn't hear. I willed one or two to look up our pathway to the window where he sat, to smile for him and wave a greeting. But my will wasn't strong enough to deliver him this small happiness, this small miracle. Passers-by were too preoccupied to see a boy at a window. In the distance I heard the wail of a police car siren. If I were curious enough I could follow the sound of the wailing siren to its destination of drama, but Barry couldn't. It was just a noise coming from nowhere and going nowhere. It and the birds and dog and shopping housewives were just brushstrokes upon the framed, contained, small canvas of his frontal vision. Each stroke separate in itself and existing for itself, with no plan or purpose or relationship.

One night, recently, I wrapped him in a blanket and took him into the back garden and let him look at the stars and moon. I'd not thought to do this before. Suddenly I wanted him to have new experiences, fill his mind with happy wonder. Things I'd always taken for granted, like moon and stars and night-sounds suddenly seemed filled with quiet and gentle magic. The moon smiled down on him, the stars gave out more luster. A kennel-tied dog mourned a sympathy from a far corner of darkness. An owl hooted a welcome . . . even the night breezes seemed to warm themselves before coming to him and touching him. I never realized, before, how much peace nighttime weaves when the looms of daytime industry are closed down and people abed and the harshness of man's reality not blaring forth from radio and television sets. Peace like a secret garden, giving off scents and perfumes from unseen flowers, filling the mind with a too rare quiet happiness. And being there with him there in the garden I suddenly felt some strange awe: an explanation of how I'd become me, explained years and years ago. How millions of sperm-seeds were sent out on a long, hard journey, millions of microscopic seeds. How, for a full-grown man to compete with that journey, he would have to cross the Sahara on foot, swim ten miles upstream against a raging current, climb the Alps and walk halfway across Siberia. . . all at one go, without pause or rest and without any help beyond his own physical resources. And if any of those seeds had reached the egg instead of my seed, I wouldn't have come into existence. . . .

And I sat with Barry and marveled that the seed that had become him had also won through; and it came to me, suddenly and startlingly, that the end of life (Barry's or my own) was not important. The miracle of everything came about with the seed's journey, which brought life into being. Sitting so with Barry, I looked at the stars and knew that we are both part of the same awesome system.

...I have learned rich things from Barry. Things I could never have learned from Bible or pulpit or churches.

I asked my wife what I must do when Barry dies.

"A handful of family," she said, "and cremate him. I can't bear to think of him being under-ground ..."

So when the time comes, open his prison and let him blow free and ride the wind and maybe, some-where, his ashes will settle and nourish the flowers.

I think of those years that I have wasted, and about people I have hurt... and I measure this, myself, against Barry's life and physically helpless existence. And I know that his has been the purer life. Everything about him exudes gentleness. He has not known hate or malice, greed or spite, or self-pity; he has not known lusts or angers, greeds or self-ishness. He has not exploded his frustrations like shrapnel to inflict wounds against those around him.

So now, when selfishness or self-pity starts to poison me, I try to think on wheelchaired Barry;

and from his helplessness, from his influence, I
find a strength and tenacity of purpose filling me up
... and then I find it no longer important to question "God's Will" but I put my trust in the Sacred
Woman, Nature, and know then that the feeling
of heartbreak in the heart of things is but a moment's human hesitation on the threshold of a deep,
serene, purposeful Unknown.

Tomorrow when sunlight has warmed our garden I shall take him down the path to the big tree.
I will show him where the squirrels live, and the
birds. The spring of the year has come home again
and spread her belongings all around. I'll show him
the flowers which grow round the tree roots, let him
take in the smells. I will let him watch spiders as
they stitch ladders ever-growing. I will let him see
the rainbows in the dewdrops ... I will let him sit
alone and at peace under the big tree, alone with
himself and the tree's life. The tree's creakings
might be conversations that he will understand in
his natural simplicity. Over the years he has
watched the tree turn to the changing seasons. He
has seen the years' leaves die and fall and has seen
each death replaced by a new birth at the spring of
each year. He has seen the buds stretch and grow
green with new life, swollen by the mother-sap's
inexhaustible goodness and richness.

I, who never knew for so many long wasted years
what love was, have learned the true richness of

what love is. Have learned from my wife and Barry. I have learned my human warmth from them—it is the community's loss that it too has not warmed its hands at the same fire.

There is a piece of music called the "Moldau" which expresses better than words what self and human integration is . . . joy, sadness, hope, love and completeness. In the music the streams and rivulets gather in the hills and the mountains, converge upon each other and increase each other, flowing on and on. The small streams wind and twist their ways round all obstacles, refusing to be stopped, and eventually the many waters form into one strong river. The river flows like a great throbbing pulse, and here and there it passes castles of enchantments, places of darknesses, it threads through sleeping villages and towns and starlit woods. The pace of the river becomes slower but more certain, much stronger; and then, finally, it joins the sea. It loses its own identity as a river, as the streams did before it, and becomes part of the greater identity, part of the sea. The Great Cosmic Intelligence.

And in the mind of man the sea is identifiable with depth, profundity, often serenity: and the sea is made up of many rivers, and the rivers in turn are made up from many streams.

Where does one identity begin and another end? The miracle is in the whole which is formed from the many parts. . . .

I look at my wife and Barry, and half-remembered lines by David Gascoyne come stumbling into my mind. . . .

> Where must I learn
> the revelation of despair, and find
> among the debris of all certainties
> the hardest stone on which to found
> altar and shelter for eternity.

A haunting magic lingers.

Postscript

CLOSED WORLD OF LOVE—so rich a world, so awesome it almost fails comprehension and denies description. How can I or anyone make words or construct sentences to describe this? Words are symbols, codes, shapes on paper. They cannot convey the heartbreak in the heart of things, they cannot show what pure unselfish love is; they can only take uncommon qualities and make them earthbound common by their sentimentality and sometimes weepiness.

I had wanted to take words and build them into a vast shining tower for my wife and her son, a beacon to outshine the brightest star . . . and cannot do it because the task is vaster than my too shallow understanding . . .